DEMYSTIFYING PANS/PANDAS

A Functional Medicine Desktop Reference
on Basal Ganglia Encephalitis

NANCY O'HARA, MD, MPH, FAAP

Published by DPWN Publishing
A division of the Dynamic Professional Women's Network, Inc.
1879 N. Neltnor Blvd. #316, West Chicago, IL 60185
www.OvercomingMediocrity.org
www.OurDPWN.com

Printed in the United States of America

ISBN: 978-1-939794-26-0

ALSO AVAILABLE:

PANS/PANDAS Clinical Membership and Mentorship with Dr. Nancy O'Hara:

- Self-paced online learning modules with brief videos and detailed lectures.

- Trademarked Functional Medicine Flow Chart.

- Monthly virtual individual and group mentoring sessions.

- Quarterly Live Q & A.

- In-office and virtual case review, troubleshooting, and examination.

Please visit www.drohara.com for more information.

Dedication and Acknowledgments

Caring for children with neurodevelopmental and neuropsychiatric illnesses has been my passion for over 25 years. It all started with one child and my introduction, during a time of my own personal infertility, to Dr. Sidney Baker: mentor and friend, one of the most brilliant men I have ever met, and the grandfather of personalized, functional medicine. I am forever grateful to him.

As with everything in caring for our children, it often takes a village. In my practice and in this guidebook, that includes my incredible and compassionate colleagues, notably Lindsey Wells, ND. I would not be able to help the children with PANS/PANDAS in our practice, continue to learn from as well as teach others, let alone remain balanced myself, without the support of my colleagues and entire staff.

I would also like to thank my co-author and wing person on this project, Sarah Ouano, ND, who has edited and co-written this guidebook with aplomb and kept me on task throughout this process. I would like to thank all the powerful and compassionate women in my life: my family, my friends, my readers, including Gabriella True, Kelly Barnhill, and Cathy Witkos, and my mom, who has always been my role model for how to live this journey with compassion and grace. Finally, I would like to thank the students and staff with whom I have worked and aided in bringing this project to fruition, particularly Shannon Wu, Yueh Qi Chuah, and Emily Walsh, for their tireless work on citations and more, and to Peter Riley on the Neurotherapy Chapter.

Finally and most essentially, I would like to thank the three most important men in my life: my father, my husband, and my son. My father has contributed immeasurably to my professional development and to this book. My husband has given me balance, perspective, and his never-ending support and unconditional love in the pursuit of all of my passions and my life. And from start to finish in my career and my life, even before he was conceived, my son. He is my inspiration and motivation for all that I do and all that I am. He is a person with more character, compassion, and strength than anyone I know. More than the gratification of my work as a doctor, mentor, and now author, I am most proud to be his mom.

Thank you.

INTRODUCTION

I've been in integrative medicine for well over twenty years. I started my career as a partner in a primary care pediatric group but had previously been a teacher of children with autism and had a great affinity for them. In my first few years of general practice, I met Noah, a four-year-old boy who presented with asthma, allergies, and autism. He was not speaking. He and his family had gone away on vacation, where he contracted a diarrheal illness. His parents called our office and spoke with the nurse, who advised them to go off dairy because the dairy might be making the diarrhea worse. He went off dairy and began talking. Once the acute illness passed, his parents incorporated dairy back into his diet, and just like that, he was once again not speaking. Noah's mom started and stopped dairy several times over the next few months, and each time, the same results. His mother called me and urged me to look further into nutrition and behavioral disorders, and at that time, I thought, "Diet change behavior? Dietary changes ameliorate Autistic symptoms? No way!" Still, the anecdotal clinical evidence was compelling, and ever the investigator, I dug in.

I was immensely fortunate at that time in my life to meet my mentor and colleague, one of the grandfathers of functional medicine: Dr. Sidney Baker. For years, I absorbed all of his teachings and the plethora of wisdom of many others. I began seeing success in caring for children with

Autism Spectrum Disorder by addressing foundational imbalances and insufficiencies, always looking for underlying infectious, immunologic, metabolic, or mitochondrial problems that they may have. I was always asking, "What does this child need that he or she is not getting?" or, "What is this child getting too much of that needs to be removed?" I was finding my stride by focusing on all of these aspects of health. Then, I met Matt. Matt presented as a ten-year-old child with a sudden onset of seizure-like tics. His family described his illness, saying, "Matt will be quietly sitting and doing homework, then thrown instantly to the ground, appearing as though he was having a seizure, his tics are so violent and progressive." In addition to these terrifying tics, he developed a sudden onset of OCD and anxiety, and his family began to see regression in his thinking and ability to complete assignments at school.

Matt was born through spontaneous vaginal delivery from a healthy pregnancy, was breastfed, and had a healthy lifestyle. He ate an organic, gluten-free, and casein-free diet. Although he had a few sensory processing issues, he was otherwise a neurotypical child. Before presenting to my office, Matt developed a viral illness with cold/upper respiratory tract symptoms. That same week, he developed a culture-positive Strep Throat and was bitten by a Lyme-positive tick. All of the bloodwork immediately following this infection was normal. Although he initially had negative Strep antibodies, these titers were elevated six weeks after his initial presentation.

In addition to these eventually positive Strep titers, we found an elevated ANA, low vitamin D, low zinc, and a positive Lyme Western blot six weeks after the infection. He was treated for three months with prescription antibiotics, then was switched to an herbal rotation of antimicrobials. During the entire course of treatment, he supplemented with zinc, vitamin D, essential fatty acids, and other natural anti-inflammatories. We also chose to incorporate helminth therapy as an alternative method of managing the autoimmune reaction and promoting immune tolerance. After three months of treatment, his tics resolved, but he was still experiencing OCD and anxiety and continued to require accommodations at school. These remaining symptoms were just attributed to "who he was," and his family learned to live with their new normal.

Years later, he presented with a "rash" that appeared as stretch marks that blanched and did not follow a normal dermal line. Instantly, I thought Bartonella, and sure enough, Matt tested positive for this Lyme co-infection. He was immediately started on a protocol of Azithromycin, Bactrim, Artemisinin, and other antimicrobial herbs, including Japanese knotweed. When these were started, his tics became much, much worse, similar to what he had experienced at age ten. Although it seems counterproductive, this abrupt flare in symptoms and even return of old symptoms is known as a Herxheimer reaction or "healing crisis," and it is not uncommon when beginning an antimicrobial protocol.

The tics continued for about six weeks after the initial onset of treatment but eventually eased, much to my relief. Interestingly, the resolution of the tics with this antibiotic and herbal protocol brought about another change—the anxiety and OCD he had been experiencing since he first presented at age ten resolved, as did the need for accommodations in school. In retrospect, I assume that he had been living with a Bartonella infection for many years, with symptoms only presenting as OCD, anxiety, and learning differences. You can read more about Matt in the case studies at the end of this guidebook.

Both Noah and Matt were keys in my learning to correctly and successfully diagnose and manage children with neurobehavioral disorders. With Noah, I learned how to support a child's health by strengthening his ability to fight disease and maintain homeostasis through diet and nutrition, in addition to appropriate therapeutic interventions. With Matt, I learned that infectious disease is multifaceted and complex and that there can be multiple culprits playing a role. I learned to always ask, as Dr. Sid had taught me, "Have we done enough for this child?" When caring for susceptible individuals, we need to create a strong foundation for health in order to build resiliency. We need to continually monitor for multiple types of infectious, autoimmune, and/or metabolic issues in order to help each child find a healthy and balanced life.

Looking back… it's almost difficult to place myself back in a time when my mind operated completely within the conventional, allopathic model. Particularly when caring for children with neurobehavioral disorders, we need more options than those available to us via the prescription pad. As Dr. Sid always reminded me: follow those who seek the truth but flee from those who have found it. Listen to each family and child to help them reach their fullest potential using a holistic and whole-child approach. I'm not here to say that every child will recover completely from whatever they have been diagnosed with, but functional medicine may be a small piece of the puzzle. It may even be a large piece of the puzzle, as it was for these children.

Being entrusted to care for these children and seeing firsthand the difference that integrative, functional medicine makes was the lightning rod that changed my way of thinking about healthcare. We have to treat the person, not the disease, and in treating the person, we have to look at the entire person, including the things that contribute to a strong foundation upon which we can build.

What is it that these children need to get? Perhaps better nutrition, cleaner air, or more potent antioxidants. What is it that these children need to get rid of? Let's consider chemical toxins, allergens, infections, and inflammation. We must investigate how each one of these aspects of health can affect an already compromised system like those of our children. I fully believe that working with children and families in an integrative, functional medicine model is the solution to this complex puzzle.

Functional Medicine: a New Frontier and Old School Wisdom

For many of us in the conventional medical world, words like "integrative," "holistic," and "natural," when linked to healthcare, can be more than a bit taboo. I was trained in the world of evidence-based practice through the example of my parents, general practitioners in my home state of West Virginia. In my youth, I believed that nutrition, herbs, and even homeopathy had no place in modern medicine because I never saw the research. The truth is, I never saw the evidence of these modalities having profound and lasting effects on the body because I wasn't looking. Working with Noah and his family inspired me to look into this world for myself, my own family, and for all the families with whom I work. My world completely opened to a new way of looking at the human body, complete with a new set of tools to complement my own skill set.

Just because I came to a mind-blowing revelation about functional medicine more than two decades ago does not mean that this concept is at all new. Naturopathic principles—seeing the body as a whole and perfect system, creating a strong foundation for health through nutrition and lifestyle, utilizing natural substances as much as possible, and teaching the patient to care for himself, to name a few!—have been documented as early as the 16th century. So much of what I practice is rooted in these concepts. While I am not a naturopathic doctor myself, I am proud to integrate my practice with naturopathic doctors, dietitians/nutritionists, and other allied health professionals because I know this approach provides the best care possible for my patients.

Many doctors and families see great success with conventional medicine alone, which is fantastic! Still, others go down the conventional route and do not see the same success. I wrote this guidebook for those families and practitioners eager to learn more but unsure of where to turn. I hope our practice and this guidebook bring the best of both of those worlds together to help each child. I want to provide a straightforward framework to diagnose, assess, and treat children with neurodevelopmental disorders, specifically PANS/PANDAS and Basal Ganglia Encephalitis. I also want to bring this debilitating but treatable disease to the forefront so that families affected by it can find a community where they feel supported and can easily seek excellent care for their children.

In true integrative style, this book is designed to help you approach a case using in-depth history taking, thorough physical examination, and conventional and functional lab testing; analyze your findings both allopathically and naturopathically; develop an individualized treatment plan that takes into account not only the diagnosis but the unique needs of each child. This is no small task, but I truly believe that once you begin to see a child through an integrative, functional medicine lens, your ability to help more families will skyrocket, and your passion for the medicine you practice will follow suit.

I am under no delusion that as a pediatrician or as a parent/caregiver of a child with neurobehavioral disorders, you have plenty of time to sit and read a textbook all about PANS/PANDAS or Basal Ganglia Encephalitis! That's why I decided to organize this book as a field guide, with straightforward chapters on the most common symptoms of PANS/PANDAS that I see, a breakdown of tests, diagnoses, and treatment options to consider for each, and a solid number of case studies for you to read through. I want you to be able to reference this book quickly during a busy workday or in small doses after your long day is complete and your children are in bed each night. Although PANS/PANDAS can be an overwhelming illness, with proper diagnosis and appropriate care, it is treatable and manageable, and I can help.

For practitioners, this book should efficiently guide you through an initial assessment, diagnosis, and treatment of a child. It will also help you know how, when, and to whom you should refer. Finally, it is meant to be the initial foundation for a mentoring relationship between you and our practice. For more information on our mentoring programs, access to lectures, videos, and live Q & A, refer to www.drohara.com. I hope to help you make your practice a place where these children and their families can heal.

Thank you for giving me the opportunity to share my hard-earned wisdom on PANS/PANDAS and Basal Ganglia Encephalitis and, more importantly, to connect with you over a topic so near and dear to me. I hope you find this book both practical and empowering and that this book and our membership and mentoring program can serve in some way as that lightning rod that unlocks a new chapter of your life.

In health,

Nancy Hofreuter O'Hara, MD, MPH, FAAP

How to Use This Desktop Reference

While the first two chapters of this book provide an overview of the history and evolution of PANS/PANDAS and Basal Ganglia Encephalitis and how to investigate these conditions properly, this book was designed to be a desktop reference instead of an exhaustive resource on the topic. I wanted to give the busy practitioner quick and easily referenced information on what can be an overwhelming topic because who has time to read a textbook while in practice?

This desktop reference is broken up into several sections—infectious agents, comorbidities and their treatments, and case studies—so that you can identify potential infection(s) at play and match comorbidities/symptoms with effective treatment options during a family's initial visit. Use the case studies to familiarize yourself with the different ways infectious and metabolic agents can manifest and learn how I would approach cases such as these.

We have listed a multitude of interventions, prescriptive as well as nutraceutical and herbal, in the following chapters. In this guidebook, we do not provide much information on specific brands or dosing, as that can be overwhelming for the child, the family, and for you. With the help of this guidebook and our membership and mentoring program, an individualized, healthy plan is achievable. We are happy to provide much more detailed and specific answers to all of your questions, including brands, dosages, and treatment methods, and to share with you our clinical knowledge and research. Please refer to www.drohara.com for more information on the mentoring and membership services offered with this guidebook.

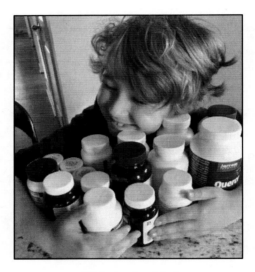

This is doable!

First Steps

It's entirely possible that you're totally new to this topic, and assessing a pediatric patient with neurobehavioral challenges is actually overwhelming. I understand! Start with the PANS/PANDAS Diagnosis Flowchart, created by the PANDAS Physicians Network (www.pandasppn.org), to orient yourself with how to assess and diagnose PANS/PANDAS. PPN is an organization dedicated to helping medical professionals better understand and care for patients with PANS/PANDAS through research and networking. You can then join our mentoring and membership program to reference the trademarked Functional Medicine PANS/PANDAS Treatment Flowchart, which we have created to include functional medicine interventions in the management of children with PANS/PANDAS and Basal Ganglia Encephalitis. Dive into the subsequent chapters to learn the major differences between PANDAS and PANS, as the two diagnoses are quite similar in every aspect except the infectious or metabolic agent triggering them.

Once you've acquainted yourself with these similar disease processes, you can begin to study the "Infectious Agents" section, which is chock full of common culprits for basal ganglia and other autoimmune encephalitis diagnoses. While they all can cause PANS/PANDAS, each infection has distinct characteristics that can be identified with physical examination, thorough history taking, and may be verified with targeted lab work.

Tailoring a Care Plan

Now, onto the "Comorbidities and their Treatments" section. I'll be honest. This is probably my favorite part of the process. Despite the fact that many cases of PANDAS and PANS can be linked to a particular infectious agent, no two children will present with the exact same symptom pattern, as each child is unique in their susceptibility and response to neuroinflammation. This section lays out most of the common symptoms that children with PANS/PANDAS and Basal Ganglia Encephalitis experience, along with treatment options from multiple branches of medicine.

Although it may seem easier to follow a treatment algorithm when you have determined a diagnosis, I have found that this does little to inspire trust and confidence from the child's family. It honestly does not yield much success in treatment. I would instead encourage you to use a patient's unique signs and symptoms to build a care plan perfectly suited to them at this particular moment in time. It is an opportunity for us to be more creative in our approach, integrating branches of medicine different from our own training and collaborating with other practitioners just down the street or across the globe.

Just some thoughts as you begin exploring the world of integrative and functional medicine to care for neurodiverse children:

- Always address inflammation. The etiology of this disease process involves inflammation in the brain, so inflammation should be addressed from the very first day, regardless of which infectious agent is involved.

- Inflammation is an autoimmune component in this disease. Investigate the patient's family history of autoimmune disease to assess the risk of autoimmunity, and create a game plan to address this as a strategy to reduce inflammation.

- Go low and slow. Some children with PANS/PANDAS tolerate aggressive treatment well, but rather than risk sending them into an exacerbation of symptoms, I recommend starting with the lowest therapeutic doses and being consistent with the treatment plan for at least one month. Discuss your approach with parents and caregivers so they can understand this and do not expect immediate results.

- Watch for multiple triggers, not forgetting about Lyme and co-infections, yeast, mold, and other bacterial or parasitic causes, especially if the onset is more subacute. Also, with a more subacute presentation, remember to delve into the history to discover if there was a previous, abrupt-onset, infection-triggered neurobehavioral event.

- Basal Ganglia Encephalitis is often an episodic course with waxing and waning symptoms, so "flares" (aggravations of symptoms) are common and normal. Prepare parents and caregivers for this and arm them with strategies to reduce flare occurrence and to minimize the intensity of flares.

- Treat the family, treat the community. If a child has a recurrence of symptoms and you suspect re-infection, look for the source in family members (including the family dog), caregivers of the child outside the home, and other community members like classmates and friend groups. Encourage those outside the home to receive effective treatment to minimize the child's exposure to infectious triggers in the future.

Your Future with PANS/PANDAS and Basal Ganglia Encephalitis

I hope this guidebook inspires you to take on patients who have been marginalized by the current healthcare system and empowers you to give them appropriate diagnoses and effective care. While the information in this book should help set you on a path to successful treatment of children with PANS/PANDAS and Basal Ganglia Encephalitis, I hope it also inspires you to dig deeper. Read the articles I reference in our extensive list of citations. Attend lectures by neurobehavioral specialists, and arrange a mentoring or membership relationship with me or someone you respect. Take a course or two on treatment techniques that you find intriguing. Let's make practicing medicine fun!

The assessment and treatment guidelines in this guidebook are mine, backed by research, nearly thirty years of clinical practice, and dozens of years of personally and professionally caring for these children and families. Read the entire guidebook sequentially or simply peruse individual chapters to help better understand, assess, and treat the children in your practice. It takes a village to care for children and families dealing with basal ganglia or other forms of autoimmune encephalitis. Thank you for allowing me to be a part of your journey.

In addition to reviewing this guidebook, if you are interested in further immersion into a functional approach to PANS/PANDAS and Basal Ganglia Encephalitis, I also offer membership subscriptions with brief videos and more detailed lectures, live Q & As, virtual mentoring, and in-person oversight. For more details, refer to www.drohara.com.

Disclaimer

The content of this guidebook is provided for informational purposes only. It is in no way intended as medical advice, a substitute for medical counseling, or as a treatment or cure for any disease or health condition. Always work with a qualified health professional before making any changes to your diet, supplement use, prescription drug use, lifestyle, or exercise activities. Readers assume all risks from the use, non-use, or misuse of the information herein.

TABLE OF CONTENTS

THE PANS/PANDAS

JOURNEY

PANS/PANDAS Integrative Treatment Flowchart[©]

Laboratory Test List

Considering PANDAS

The Introduction of PANS

Note: further guidance on treatment, including dosages and preferred brands, is available through membership and mentorship options at www.drohara.com

PANS/PANDAS Integrative Treatment Flowchart©

For practitioner access to the full resolution Integrative Treatment Flowchart, please register your name and credentials at www.drohara.com.

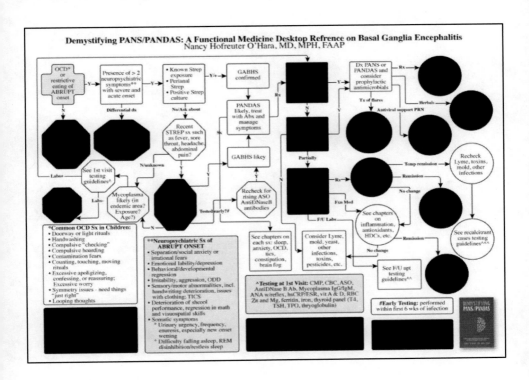

Demystifying PANS/PANDAS: A Functional Medicine Desktop Refrence on Basal Ganglia Encephalitis
Nancy Hofreuter O'Hara, MD, MPH, FAAP

LABORATORY TEST LIST

As you may know, PANS, PANDAS, and Basal Ganglia Encephalitis are clinical diagnoses. While laboratory evaluation is helpful to determine an infectious cause, nutrient deficiency, inflammation, or other factors impacting a child's symptoms, they are not diagnostic. Please consider the following lists to guide your evaluation at the initial consultation and beyond.

Labs to Consider at Initial Consultation

- CMP (complete metabolic panel, including liver and kidney function)
- CBC, with differential and platelets
- ANA with reflex panel
- hs-CRP
- ESR
- ASO
- AntiDNaseB antibody
- Mycoplasma IgG and IgM, consider IFA
- TSH, T4, and thyroid antibodies (TPO, thyroglobulin)
- RBC zinc, magnesium

- Iron, ferritin

- 25-hydroxyvitamin D

- Vitamin A

Additional Tests (Depending on History and Physical Examination)

- IgA and IgG subclasses

- Strep pneumococcal serotypes (14-23)

- Ionized calcium

- Selenium (red blood cell, if possible)

- Molybdenum

- Mitochondrial markers (CK, carnitine, acylcarnitine profile, ammonia, lactate, plasma amino acids looking specifically at alanine (> 450 or alanine: lysine ratio > 2.5) and vitamin B12 levels, which should be measured via an MMA, methylmalonic acid (high MMA consistent with a low intracellular B12)

- Viral titers, including MMR, varicella, HHV6, HSV, EBV, and CMV

Specialty Labs to Consider

- MTHFR and other SNPs

- OAT (Urine Organic Acid Test)

- Stool analysis: CDSA (Comprehensive Digestive Stool Analysis) or local stool mycology, microbiology, and parasitology

- Lyme and co-infections (especially Bartonella and Babesia), including specialty lab testing

- Mold (ERMI, urine mycotoxins, and other markers)

For more details on laboratory testing and interpretation, please see the videos in our membership program at www.drohara.com.

Considering PANDAS

If you're reading this book, you probably know someone affected by PANS/PANDAS, or you are a practitioner with some experience in caring for children with neurodevelopmental disorders and are interested in knowing more about it. I say this with certainty because PANS/PANDAS is a bit of a controversial diagnosis—many people have never heard of it, and most medical institutions teach nothing about it. An unfortunate side effect of this is that families affected by PANS/PANDAS struggle to receive a proper diagnosis. Therefore, treatment of the disease and resources to help these families are few and far between. In fact, more than 60% of my patients consulted with more than three practitioners before they were correctly diagnosed.[1] I desperately want to change this, and I'm sure you do, too.

When children present with abrupt onset of behavioral changes, it affects the entire family.[2] Wraparound services for both the parents and siblings of our children with PANS/PANDAS are extremely important to the success of our treatments, but it truly does start with diagnosis. If you can learn to diagnose this disease process clinically, you will become a valued resource in your community. This chapter will outline the assessment, diagnosis, and treatment of children with PANDAS and those with PANS in the next chapter. You will see the clinical presentation and symptoms are often the same; both fall under the categorization of Basal Ganglia Encephalitis.

So, What is PANDAS?

Pediatric Autoimmune Neuropsychiatric Disorders Associated with Streptococcal infections, or PANDAS, is an abrupt-onset infectious and immunologic disease subset within the pediatric population, typically observed between ages three and puberty, but can present in adolescence and even adulthood.[3] Diagnoses made later in childhood or adulthood are sometimes caused by a previous misdiagnosis and, in these cases, may be more sub-acute in their presentations. I am writing this guidebook and providing this mentorship to prevent this, as it is vital to recognize and treat this disorder as early as possible. I urge all practitioners to assess for infection-triggered diseases whenever a child presents with an abrupt onset of neuropsychiatric symptoms. In other words, obtain a Strep culture and initiate a detailed history prior to starting an SSRI or other conventional psychiatric intervention.

A child may be diagnosed with PANDAS when Obsessive-Compulsive Disorder (OCD), tic disorder, or both suddenly appear following a Streptococcal (Strep) infection, such as Strep throat, rectal Strep, or scarlet fever. This devastating but treatable autoimmune disease has been found in approximately one in 200 children. It results from immune cells attacking the basal ganglia in the brain in a molecular mimicry battle against Strep.

There are multiple studies demonstrating autoimmunity and Strep-specific immune activation, as below:

- Strep-specific TH17 lymphocytes open BBB in mouse models.[4]

- Strep auto-antibodies are shown to cross-react in Basal Ganglia Encephalitis.[5]

- Studies have identified cerebral microstructural differences in children with PANS, especially the deep gray matter, including the thalamus, basal ganglia, and amygdala.[6]

- In addition to summarizing and analyzing the research on structural CNS findings of the caudate, putamen, globus pallidus, and striatum, the presence of autoantibodies interacting with the basal ganglia and the genetic predispositions, a recent study by Baj et al., further provided insight into alterations to the gut microbiota in children with PANDAS.[7]

- Structural and functional features of CNS Lymphatic channels link the immune system and brain.[8]

- Intranasal Group A Strep promotes CNS infiltration of TH17 cells.[9]

You may see children in your practice with some symptoms of OCD or tics, with low intensity and minimal side effects, with subacute or chronic presentations, and you should suspect that these children do not fall into a PANDAS diagnosis (unless they have historically exhibited a previous abrupt onset of these symptoms). When there is a true onset of PANDAS, there is a significant change from their everyday worries and sensory challenges, and the development is typically quite rapid. Literally, these symptoms come from out of nowhere and often overnight!

Many parents can tell you the date and time their child started exhibiting these often shocking and upsetting symptoms. PANS/PANDAS, also appropriately termed autoimmune encephalitis of the basal ganglia or Basal Ganglia Encephalitis (BGE), includes:

- An ABRUPT, dramatic onset or recurrence of OCD, acute-onset anorexia, and/or severe, restrictive eating disorders.

- Concurrent presence of additional behavioral or neurologic symptoms with similarly acute onset and severity from at least TWO of the following categories:

  o Anxiety, including separation anxiety (at bedtime, school, not wanting to leave parent's side), is often accompanied by a hyper-alert appearance ("deer in headlights").

  o Behavioral/developmental regression (baby talk, tantrums, suddenly playing with younger siblings or acquaintances).

  o Emotional lability/emotional regression, including suicidal depression and hallucinations of any sort.

  o Irritability, aggression, raging, self-injurious behaviors, and/or severe oppositional behaviors.

  o Sensory or motor abnormalities, including visuospatial and handwriting deterioration, tics, hypersensitivity, or insensitivity, sometimes with physical examination findings of choreiform movements of hands ("piano-playing" fingers).

  o Deterioration in school performance and cognitive changes (new and abrupt changes in grades, attention, testing, onset of ADHD or hyperactivity, inability to concentrate, decreased processing speed, or executive function differences).

  o Somatic signs and symptoms.

    ▪ Sleep disturbances (difficulty falling asleep, REM disinhibition/restless sleep, night terrors, refusal to sleep alone).

    ▪ Urinary frequency or urgency, including increased daytime "accidents" or new-onset enuresis.

o Symptoms are not better explained by another known neurologic or medical disorder.

It is interesting to note how frequently these symptoms appear in PANDAS-affected children. Eating disorders appear in only 20% of Basal Ganglia Encephalitis cases, while 60% of children report aggression and acute onset of learning disorder, 70% experience hyperactivity and tics, 80% exhibit a hyper-alert appearance, up to 85% have shown REM disinhibition on sleep study, 90% have difficulty concentrating, have urinary changes, or display handwriting deterioration, and 98% experience separation anxiety.[10]

In other research papers, the numbers have fluctuated somewhat. For example, in a 2015 paper in JCAP, researchers found differences in the clinical vs. research setting: 67% of children displayed tics from a research setting versus 60% in a community setting; and for hyperactivity, 92% and 47%, respectively.[11]

While every child is unique, there are clear hallmarks of this disease, and our children cannot afford for us to remain uneducated about them.

Investigating PANDAS

Suppose your patient or child is between the ages of 3 and 13, or even if they are older, and has an abrupt or dramatic change of behavioral symptoms, particularly neurologic abnormalities (such as motoric hyperactivity, choreiform movements, and separation anxiety). In that case, you must start investigating PANDAS immediately. Keep in mind that PANDAS is a **clinical** diagnosis only, so although we have many diagnostic tests at our disposal to consider, these only build a case for PANDAS rather than confirm or deny its existence. It is also important to remember that PANDAS has an episodic course of symptom severity—waxing and waning of symptoms is normal and even expected to some degree after the initial presentation.

Patient Interview

The patient interview and discussions with parents are key in gathering appropriate information necessary to make a PANS/PANDAS diagnosis. Parents may first report an increase in a child going to the bathroom. Further questioning may reveal that this is caused by the emergence of OCD symptoms, including excessive hand washing, wanting to dress and undress, or simply anxiety. Many children with OCD may have intrusive thoughts and mental compulsions. These children try very hard to hide these intrusive thoughts. As practitioners, we may not easily identify physical compulsions or even see these intrusive thoughts as mental compulsions. It is important to listen, look, and identify all of these Obsessive-Compulsive Disorders (see OCD Chapter).

Parents may also report behavioral regression or "baby talk," social regression with wanting to spend time with younger children, or separation anxiety. There can be changes in energy levels—hyperactivity or exhaustion—caused by new sleep issues. They may also suggest a loss of executive function, seen with an abrupt onset of increased disorganization, problems with decision making, time management, attention, and following directions.

Additional symptoms caregivers may report include abrupt onset of:

- Shortened attention span
- Difficulty with memory
- Loss of math visuospatial skills

- Clumsiness
- Executive function deficits
- Tics or choreiform movements
- Elevated OCD and anxiety in test situations

Family History

Take an in-depth family history to determine a child's risk of PANDAS. Because of the autoimmune component of the disease, it is unsurprising that we find a significant connection between patients with PANDAS and a strong family history of autoimmune disease. In our practice, over 60% of children with PANS/PANDAS have a first-degree relative with autoimmune disease, including autoimmune thyroiditis, inflammatory bowel disease, arthritis, diabetes, or a family history of rheumatic fever, among others.

Physical Examination

A thorough physical examination can also give greater insight into the presence of PANDAS. Some children may present with the classic "strawberry tongue" of Strep. Some may have peeling fingers and toes, sometimes seen up to six weeks post-Strep infection. Both are pictured below.

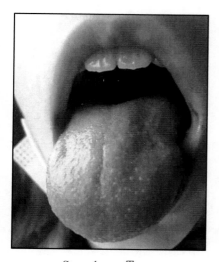

Strawberry Tongue

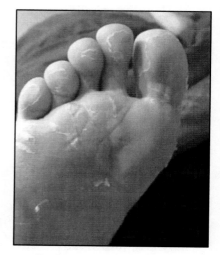

*Peeling Toes Six Weeks After
Strep Infection*

You may also find the following during the physical exam:

- Hyper-alertness with dilated pupils

- Red ring around the anus (seen with rectal Strep)

- Scarlatina rash

- Damaged nail bed vasculature

- Palatal petechiae

- Throat findings including erythema, purulence, enlarged tonsils

- Cervical adenopathy

- Choreiform movements ("piano-playing fingers") as described below

Choreiform movements are tiny involuntary movements that may appear similar to piano-playing fingers and/or supination of hands when trying to hold them steady. These movements are indicative of brain inflammation and a diagnostic sign of Basal Ganglia Encephalitis, PANS, and PANDAS. In your office or your description to parents, have the child stand upright with feet together, arms outstretched, elbows straight, and fingers spread wide. Then ask the child to shut their eyes. Stand near them in case they become unsteady. A child should be able to stand still without hand or finger movements for at least 30-60 seconds. With inflammation of the basal ganglia and when a child is in a flare, they will not be able to hold their fingers and/or hands steady. Instead, the fingers start to move as if they were playing the piano subtly or more significantly, and/or hands roll outward in a supinating manner (please refer to our videos of the physical exam and specifically these choreiform movements at www.drohara.com).

You can also instruct parents to use this technique at times of increased behaviors, rage, anxiety, OCD, or tics. If the child can not hold steady and these movements are evident, then that indicates that the symptoms are part of an inflammatory flare and should be treated with Ibuprofen or similar anti-inflammatories. Their practitioner should be notified immediately.

Note that it is also possible that you uncover no physical signs at all!

Laboratory Testing

PANDAS is associated with Group A beta-hemolytic Streptococcal infection, which can be determined through a positive throat culture for Strep, a reported history of scarlet fever, or sometimes an anal/rectal culture of Strep. However, some Strep infections are not so clear-cut. Sometimes, you will only have intimate exposure to Group A Strep and subsequent behavioral changes. Blood antibody tests may or may not be positive. Although Strep is most likely to be found in the throat, it may also be found in the tonsils, adenoids, sinuses, skin with severe eczema or psoriasis, and in the urinary, vaginal, or GI tract. Rectal swabs may uncover an underlying Strep infection when a blood antibody test and throat swab reveal nothing. Keep in mind, too, that the tonsils are a challenging area to diagnose, as surface microbes of the tonsils may differ greatly from those in the tonsillar core. In short, due to poor technique, an uncooperative child, or lack of appropriate culture (e.g., only performing a rapid Strep), the throat culture may be negative. You may not appropriately identify these germs until a tonsillectomy is performed, so the culture of these tissues during tonsillectomy and adenoidectomy is essential. More on that later.

Consider checking family members as well. Take cultures of all parents, caregivers, siblings, and even the family dog if necessary. Although the child does not need to be actively fighting Strep in order to trigger PANDAS (even exposure at school or day camp is sufficient to set off the sequelae of this disease), it is important to address Strep infections, to check cultures, and possibly titers where indicated, in all those the child comes into frequent contact with if possible.

Keep in mind that although the laboratory tests listed below may be helpful, they neither confirm nor deny the diagnosis. To make the diagnosis of PANDAS, you only need the abrupt onset of neurobehavioral symptoms listed above, in conjunction with a Strep infection or Strep in an intimate contact in the preceding 6-12 weeks. Reference the Laboratory Testing Guidelines for additional considerations.

In our clinical practice, the most commonly positive lab marker is ANA, found in almost 60% of our patients. Chang et al. noted that up to 13% of healthy children might demonstrate a nonspecific positive ANA.[12]

Essential Tests to Order

- Culture of possible infectious sites: Strep and viral cultures

- Inflammatory markers: CRP, ESR, ANA (> 56 % +)[13]

- Infectious markers: ASO, antiDNaseB Ab, Mycoplasma IgG, IgM (six weeks after infection; do NOT treat titers)

Additional Tests to Consider

- Mitochondrial markers (carnitine, acylcarnitine, ammonia, lactic acid, and creatinine kinase), especially if the child has low tone, constipation, or another of the myriad of signs indicating mitochondrial dysfunction. Mitochondrial dysfunction can occur secondary to any significant infectious or autoimmune disorder and should be considered if such symptoms are present.

- Mineral levels should be evaluated within the red blood cells, as RBC measurements give us a more accurate representation of intracellular levels. We especially consider zinc, magnesium, and iron (with ferritin level, both as a reflection of iron stores and, if elevated, as an acute phase reactant) and usually add calcium (ionized), selenium, and molybdenum.

- Thyroid markers T4, TSH, and thyroid antibodies, including thyroid peroxidase (TPO) antibody and thyroglobulin antibody.

- Antioxidants, especially vitamins A and D

- Viral titers, especially Measles, Mumps, Rubella, and Varicella, as well as Herpes and EBV/CMV if these are considered triggers for a child.

- Immunoglobulins, including IgG and subclasses, and Strep pneumococcal serotypes if immunodeficiency is considered.

- Methylation analysis may include homocysteine, cysteine, and MTHFR, as this genetic defect (particularly defects in C677 allele) can affect folate metabolism and, therefore, methylation.

Analysis

When considering PANDAS, it is important to rule out other disease processes with similar abrupt onset, including:

- Other forms of encephalitis and cerebral vasculitis[14]

- Child abuse, sexual abuse, or psychological or other trauma or head injury

- Exposure to toxins, medications, or illicit drugs

- Tumors and strokes

- Sydenham chorea associated with rheumatic fever

As you know, Tourette's and OCD do not typically feature an acute onset, so it should not be part of the initial differential if an accurate history is obtained. Most of the above abrupt onset diseases can be diagnosed by history and physical exam. Still, tests such as CT or MRI, EEG, and CSF analysis should be considered and obtained as appropriate.

Treatment

Treatment for PANDAS should include a three-pronged approach:

1. Reduce the incidence and severity of symptoms with a tailored plan of care, including therapy (CBT), supplements/ nutraceuticals, and possibly psychoactive medications.

2. Kill the pathogen to remove the infection/source of inflammation.

3. Provide ongoing immunomodulation to treat and manage inflammation.

Most physicians can agree that when we see an infection, the obvious solution is to administer an antibiotic to eradicate it. PANDAS treatment is no different. Antimicrobials, whether pharmaceutical or herbal, are a crucial step in effectively managing PANDAS. In the acute situation and with abrupt onset, I almost universally begin with a three to four-week course of antibiotics, as these are research-proven and tend to work quickly. The most common pharmaceutical antibiotics used are: Azithromycin, Penicillin, Amoxicillin-Clavulanate, Clarithromycin, Cephalexin, Cefadroxil, Cefdinir, and Clindamycin, and I usually start with Azithromycin, Cefdinir, or Amoxicillin-Clavulanate.

I also find great success with utilizing antimicrobial herbs with PANDAS children, including:

- Berberine, a constituent found in *Hydrastis Canadensis* (goldenseal), prevents the adherence of Strep to body cells and prevents the synthesis of Strep DNA.[15]

- *Azadirachta indica*, Neem, is a gentle but powerful Ayurvedic herb used in many natural toothpastes for its ability to inhibit the growth of four Streptococcus strains associated with dental caries formation.[16] It can be used to manage both Strep and *Candida albicans*.

- *Usnea barbata*, or beard moss, is a medicinal lichen used since ancient times as an antibiotic. It has shown to be effective against gram-positive bacteria[17] such as Streptococcus,[18] Staphylococcus (impetigo, etc.), *Mycobacterium tuberculosis*, and other fast-growing species.

At the onset of treatment, PANDAS symptoms can temporarily worsen as the body wages war on the offending pathogen. Those familiar with naturopathic medicine might know this as a "healing crisis," while others in the Lyme-literate community call it a Herxheimer's reaction. The die-off caused by aggressive antibiotic treatment, whether pharmaceutical or herbal, can certainly make the child feel temporarily worse, so symptom management is an equally important aspect of effective PANDAS care. These supportive interventions are as unique as your patient, so tailor your care plan according to individual symptoms. You'll find treatment recommendations for common symptoms in each of the symptom chapters and more on the Herxheimer reaction in the Lyme chapter. Often with the initiation of antibiotic treatment, there is improvement in symptoms, and this is not just therapeutic but also diagnostic of PANDAS.

As discussed in other chapters, even if you can not determine the exact infectious trigger, JCAP guidelines recommend an extended course of antibiotics to treat Strep. We also recommend this for those with identified Mycoplasma and other infectious triggers such as Lyme, Babesia, and Bartonella, as outlined in those chapters. After initial effective treatment, continued prophylactic antibiotics or antimicrobials must be considered. This effective treatment prototype was first outlined in the treatment and prophylaxis of rheumatic fever and Sydenham chorea.[19]

In addition to managing healing crises, we must focus on the symptoms which are causing the most issues for a child. Examples of this include using a sleep aid or sleep hygiene to improve sleep, using adaptogens to decrease anxiety or OCD by helping the child build resilience to adrenal stress, or using mitochondrial support to aid fatigue or cognitive issues. This guidebook includes several chapters on these symptoms and appropriate interventions to consider.

The last essential component of effective PANDAS treatment is to decrease inflammation and modulate the immune system to prevent an inappropriate response in the future. While a good deal of inflammation can be addressed with antibiotic use alone, it is oftentimes necessary to include other immunomodulating pharmaceuticals or long-term anti-inflammatory substances to keep inflammation at bay. Most commonly, I utilize probiotics, herbal anti-inflammatories, essential fatty acids, antioxidant vitamins, helminths, or prescriptive steroids for this purpose. In moderate or more severe cases, IVIG may be considered, and plasmapheresis or monoclonal antibodies may be needed.

For further information, refer to subsequent sections on antimicrobials, inflammation, and treatment of symptoms. For details on dosages and specifics on treatments, refer to our membership and mentoring program at www.drohara.com.

Therapy as Diagnosis

As I mentioned previously, treatment for PANDAS can also serve as a diagnostic tool. Ibuprofen, for instance, is an excellent anti-inflammatory medication, and it is safe to administer up to 10 milligrams per kilogram every 6 to 8 hours for short-term relief. If a child's symptoms improve with Ibuprofen, it may indicate that their symptoms (anxiety, tics, agitation, OCD) are triggered by inflammation, and longer-term immunotherapy may be helpful.[20]

Like Ibuprofen, prescription steroids can also be used therapeutically, as well as diagnostically. If a child improves with a short course of steroids, an inflammatory reaction is highly likely, and a need for further therapy, such as IVIG, may be indicated.

I strongly encourage a trial of antibiotics and Ibuprofen at the first sign of acute onset symptoms. If inflammation is at all at play, there will be a marked improvement with these safe and inexpensive medications and will buy the practitioner time to develop a more tailored treatment plan.

The PANDAS Controversy

When speaking to people about this epidemic, you may start to see their eyes glaze over. It's not an easy thing to understand. You may hear, "I don't get it. Is it Lyme or Strep, and how does that explain why your kid is freaking out on this play date because you just walked out of the room?!" Honestly, most people unaffected by PANDAS just won't get it. The truth is that PANS and PANDAS cases have been present for decades but was rarely diagnosed accurately, so these diseases are not well known or understood by most people. Hopefully, the identification of this diagnosis is on the rise.

Various studies have found that 79% of pediatricians will treat presumed Strep with antibiotics without a positive culture.[21] For example, if you take Johnny to the pediatrician because he is complaining about a sore throat and may also have a sinus or ear infection, the doctor may put him on antibiotics without ever confirming he had Strep. Fast forward to two months later when PANDAS symptoms abruptly appear, and there is no documented history of Strep. Now, these symptoms are considered a behavioral or psychological issue rather than what they are: abrupt-onset of neurological manifestations of an infectious and inflammatory disease. The second issue that arises in this scenario is that if Johnny is treated with Amoxicillin several times in his lifetime and then is suspected of having PANDAS, treatment with Amoxicillin alone might not help the symptoms, as he may now be resistant. Being open to a trial of antibiotics with the abrupt onset of the above neurobehavioral symptoms is the first step to turning this devastating illness into a treatable disorder.

Limited "Evidence"

Although there are currently multiple studies investigating PANDAS, only a small number of prospective studies exist. Studies are mostly conducted retrospectively, which limits how much information we have at any moment to confirm what we see in clinical practice. There is also ambiguity and skepticism in establishing a group A Strep relatedness to OCD, tics, and other symptoms. However, several studies have shown that children with OCD and tics were more likely than the control group to have prior Strep infections over three months before the onset of symptoms and even more likely to have multiple Strep infections within 12 months before the onset of symptoms. More confirmatory research is needed, but the evidence is not scarce. [22, 23, 24, 25]

As you can see from the average number of doctors that parents consult before receiving a proper diagnosis, we have our work cut out for us in terms of spreading awareness and educating more medical providers that PANDAS is real and worth our attention. Too many children are languishing with insufficient and incorrect care. Thank you for being a part of the solution in the education and awareness of PANDAS; now, let's get to work.

The Introduction of PANS

In 1998, Dr. Sue Swedo first proposed PANDAS (Pediatric Autoimmune Neuropsychiatric Disorders Associated with Strep) to explain an association between Strep throat and obsessive-compulsive and tic disorders.[26] According to her report, an immune response to Group A *Streptococcus (GAS) pyogenes* infection triggered a host of psychiatric complications. In 2012, together with thirty other practitioners, researchers, and colleagues, she revised her criteria to include additional causes of autoimmune encephalitis, and Pediatric Acute-onset Neuropsychiatric Syndromes (PANS) was officially presented as a diagnosis.[27] The definition of PANS includes infectious causes other than Strep, such as Mycoplasma and viruses, as well as environmental causes like anesthesia, pesticides, and chemicals.

Diagnostic Criteria

Diagnosing PANS follows the same process as that of PANDAS and, by definition, includes:

- An ABRUPT, dramatic onset or recurrence of OCD, acute-onset anorexia, and/or severe, restrictive eating disorders

- Concurrent presence of additional behavioral or neurologic symptoms with similarly acute onset and severity from at least TWO of the following categories:

o Anxiety, including separation anxiety (at bedtime, school, not wanting to leave parent's side) often accompanied by a hyper-alert appearance ("deer in the headlights").

o Behavioral/developmental regression (baby talk, tantrums, suddenly playing with younger siblings or acquaintances).

o Emotional lability/emotional regression, including suicidal depression and hallucinations of any sort.

o Irritability, aggression, raging, self-injurious behaviors, and/or severe oppositional behaviors.

o Sensory or motor abnormalities, including tics and deterioration of handwriting, hypersensitivity, or insensitivity, sometimes with physical examination findings of choreiform movements of hands ("piano-playing" fingers).

o Deterioration in school performance and cognitive changes (new and abrupt changes in grades, attention, and testing, abrupt onset of ADHD or hyperactivity, inability to concentrate, decreased processing speed, or executive function differences).

o Somatic signs and symptoms

  ▪ Sleep disturbances (difficulty falling asleep, REM disinhibition/restless sleep, night terrors, refusal to sleep alone).

  ▪ Urinary frequency or urgency, including increased daytime "accidents" or new-onset enuresis.

o Symptoms are not better explained by another known neurologic or medical disorder.

Similar to PANDAS, PANS is a clinical diagnosis confirmed with or without laboratory evidence. Clinicians should confirm PANS by investigating Strep titers (ASO and anti-DNase B Ab), inflammatory markers, and infectious disease testing (especially Mycoplasma as well as viruses, Lyme, and mold). Treatment with antimicrobials and immune modulators can be used as a diagnostic tool as well as a therapeutic intervention. If financially feasible for caregivers, I also like to include a urine organic acid test (OAT) to determine any metabolic abnormalities. This test gives skilled practitioners insight into potential infections, as it measures the metabolites of certain organisms. It can also tell us much about a child's detoxification mechanisms, oxidative stress levels, and nutrient stores.

Refer to the PANDAS chapter for a list of testing to consider. As for antibiotics, if Mycoplasma is suspected or endemic in your area, consider initial use of Azithromycin, as this will treat Mycoplasma in addition to Strep (review local resistance in your area). In addition to antibiotics that treat Mycoplasma (namely, Macrolides and Tetracyclines), natural products, such as Berberine (as from Goldenseal), Houttuynia, Isatis, and colloidal silver (also good for Strep) may be considered.

Treating PANS

Early and accurate diagnosis and treatment result in better outcomes. It is important that we do not blame the family or the child for the behavioral changes, as this is truly an infectious and immunologic disease at play. We must reassure parents that their children can get better but may need some accommodations in school and at home.

The approach to the treatment of PANS, like PANDAS, is three-pronged:

- Treat the symptoms

- o Cognitive Behavioral Therapy (CBT); consider Exposure and Response Prevention (ERP) and Dialectical Behavioral Therapy (DBT).

- o Supplements, adaptogens, and antioxidant/metabolic support

- o Psychoactive medications such as SSRIs and SNRIs (start low and go slow, remembering that some children may experience adverse reactions).

- Remove the source of the inflammation

  - o Antimicrobials/antibiotics, both therapeutic and prophylactic

  - o Antivirals and antioxidants, if viruses are the suspected source of infection.

  - o Watch for signs of a "healing crisis," Herxheimer reaction, or die-off, and see the chapter on Lyme for more information on this.

- Treat immune disturbances with immunomodulators and/or anti-inflammatories determined by symptom severity

  - o Anti-inflammatory nutraceuticals, NSAIDs (Ibuprofen), and corticosteroids

  - o Intravenous Immunoglobulin (IVIG)

  - o Plasmapheresis (PEX)/Therapeutic Plasma Exchange (TPE)

  - o Monoclonal Antibodies, Rituximab, Cellcept, and other immunomodulatory agents.

Other Treatment Options

We go into greater detail about treatment in the "Comorbidities and Their Treatments" section of this book, as well as when to apply each, depending on the severity of the presentation. However, below is a brief overview of some generalized interventions that we might employ and may not otherwise be discussed in subsequent chapters.

1. Tonsillectomy and adenoidectomy (T&A): Published research regarding the therapeutic benefit of tonsillectomy and autoimmune encephalitis is mixed. In clinical practice, we see improvement in at least 50% of these patients, particularly those with PANDAS (Strep). In fact, many children who would benefit from this treatment have damaged or cryptic tonsils, although this is not the only time when tonsillectomy may be indicated. In an unpublished study performed at Georgetown University, researchers found that tonsils belonging to patients with PANDAS contained elevated levels of Th17, suggesting a sustained immune response in this localized area. For those unfamiliar, Th17 is an agent allowing inflammation in targeted regions of the brain. We are finding that removal of chronically inflamed and infected tissue can dramatically reduce, if not eliminate, PANS/PANDAS symptoms when combined with wraparound care.[28] Tonsillectomy/adenoidectomy is definitely recommended in those children with other reasons for removal, such as chronic/recurrent Strep infections or sleep apnea. Essential during T & A is the culture of the tissue, as these can be discordant between surface and core pathogens. Appropriate culture can better guide care.

   Given the somewhat controversial nature of T&A, I outline several recent studies below for your consideration:

   - Navin et al. reports that "caregivers reported a decreasing frequency of symptoms over time, regardless of treatment, and had no difference in satisfaction. T&A was the most preferred treatment and the most impactful on symptoms for surgical patients. Given the challenges of immunologic therapies, T&A in combination with antibiotics should be considered as an early intervention for PANDAS."[29]

- Demesh et al. writes that "although the current evidence is inconclusive, the data reported herein support previously described smaller case series and further strengthens the notion that tonsillectomy may benefit patients with PANDAS whose symptoms are not controlled with antibiotic therapy." One caveat to this study would be subject recall bias, as information was extracted retrospectively from the parents' historical accounts of symptoms using a non-validated symptom severity score.[30]

- A study conducted by Pavone et al. in 2014 included 120 patients with PANDAS, followed for 24 months, who either had undergone T&A or had been managed conservatively. There was no difference in the two groups between clinical progression, antibody production, or neuropsychiatric symptoms.[31]

- Two case studies (one by Alexander and another by Hubi) both showed positive results from T & A.[32, 33]

- Murphy et al. played a crucial role in refuting the notion that tonsillectomy may play a protective role in the development of the disease.[34]

- Finally, Amarkumar reviewed the literature to date, concluding that the literature was limited in providing definitive conclusions and that prospective study was further required.

2. Antihistamines: pharmaceutical antihistamines are excellent anti-inflammatory and immunomodulatory agents. Still, they may also have the added benefit of being sedative (such as Diphenhydramine), which can benefit children with PANS/PANDAS—induced sleep disturbances. Be aware that antihistamines have the potential for a paradoxical reaction in some children, so they should be closely monitored and started on low doses to ensure safety.

3. School-based interventions: oftentimes, some of the anxiety a child experiences, is rooted in issues or fears about school or with school routines and rules. Because PANDAS, PANS, and Basal Ganglia Encephalitis are medical diagnoses, schools should comply with accommodations with a practitioner's request or statement. Both parents and practitioners should be knowledgeable about how their local school systems can help children with PANS/PANDAS during active exacerbations of their conditions (what we call "flares"). Consider the following to reduce symptoms and promote normalcy as needed in each individual case:

    a. Low key access to the bathroom

    b. Late passes on file at school to allow for later starts and excused absences.

    c. Home study options

    d. Shortened school days or weeks

    e. Adaptive physical education

    f. Use of assisted technology to work around dysgraphia (handwriting deterioration).

g. Additional time granted for homework, in-school assignments, tests, and getting to class.

4. IVIG: Intravenous immunoglobulin (IVIG) is an expensive intervention that utilizes a blood product prepared from the serum of blood donors. It is a highly effective treatment for patients with antibody deficiencies, as it interferes with the emergence of B cells from the bone marrow and controls B and T cell proliferation. It neutralizes auto antibodies and bacterial toxins and guides immune cells to act more appropriately. When caring for a child with PANDAS, high doses (1.5-2 g/kg) may be necessary to reverse the autoimmune response. It is now recognized that up to 6 monthly cycles may be needed to gain traction on treating the autoimmune effects of PANS/PANDAS.[35] However, if the child also has an immune deficiency, lower doses (400-600 mg/kg) may be initiated at first. Be aware that in some cases, low-dose treatment may exacerbate neurobehavioral symptoms, so consultation with an immunologist is imperative when this treatment is indicated. Please refer to the chapter on Inflammation for further information on IVIG and when it may be appropriate.

5. Plasmapheresis and monoclonal antibodies:

a. In severe cases, Plasmapheresis (PEX), also termed Therapeutic Plasma Exchange (TPE) or Therapeutic Plasma Apheresis (TPA), may generate the fastest and most significant improvement. It has been proposed as a potential treatment for severe cases of Basal Ganglia Encephalitis because of its success in treating Sydenham chorea. Latimer et al. performed a retrospective review of all PANDAS patients treated with TPA at Georgetown University Hospital between August 2009 and October 2013: "All patients were reported to have received at least some benefit from TPA, with an average improvement of 65% at six months post-TPA and 78% at longer-term follow-up. A decrease in the number of reported symptoms also occurred, with particular improvements in obsessive-compulsive disorder (OCD), anxiety, tics, and somatic symptoms, including dysgraphia, sleep difficulties, and urinary urgency or frequency. Contrary to expectations, preceding duration of illness was not correlated with the degree of improvement following TPA."[36]

b. Rituximab is a monoclonal antibody that binds the surface protein CD-20, widely expressed on B-lymphocytes. It triggers cell death and has been used in the last 20 years for several lymphoid malignancies. Because of its positive effects on auto-immune and dys-immunological diseases, it has gained attention also for psychiatric disorders with a probable immunological etiology. Given the evidence about a possible role of inflammation in OCD pathophysiology, Rituximab is now considered in the treatment of severe cases of PANS/PANDAS.[37] Please refer to the chapter on Inflammation for further information on plasmapheresis, IV monoclonal antibody therapy, and when these may be indicated.

In addition to the treatment modalities listed above and in coming chapters, it is essential to understand the interventions based on symptom severity. Despite the success rate in helping children recover from PANS and PANDAS, it should be noted that these interventions can be highly cost-prohibitive, often not covered by private insurance, and require specialists well versed in them. Therefore, I encourage practitioners to become educated about the plethora of other treatments available to their patients, outlined in the coming chapters, in order to find an attainable path to healing for families.

MEET THE INFECTIOUS AGENTS

Group A Streptococcus and PANDAS

Mycoplasma and PANS

Viruses

Yeast Dysbiosis

Mold and Chronic Inflammatory Response Syndrome (CIRS)

Other Infections: Parasites, Clostridia, Lyme Disease, and Co-infections

Note: further guidance on treatment, including dosages and preferred brands, is available through membership and mentorship options at <u>www.drohara.com</u>.

GROUP A STREPTOCOCCUS AND PANDAS

In 1998, Dr. Sue Swedo first proposed PANDAS (Pediatric Autoimmune Neuropsychiatric Disorders Associated with Strep) in her seminal paper to explain an association between Strep throat and obsessive-compulsive and tic disorders. According to Dr. Swedo, an immune response to Group A Streptococcus infection triggered a host of psychiatric complications, including anxiety, tics, OCD, and emotional lability.[38] The symptoms of PANDAS reflected many of the symptoms described with Sydenham chorea (SC) decades earlier. With SC, it had been previously shown that 95% of these children had emotional lability and up to 75% at initial presentation, and 100% with recurrence had OCD.[39]

Strep Basics

Streptococcus pyogenes is responsible for a host of disease states, including pharyngitis (Strep throat), scarlet fever, impetigo, type II necrotizing fasciitis, cellulitis, Streptococcal toxic shock syndrome, acute rheumatic fever, post-Streptococcal glomerulonephritis, and of course, PANDAS. Strep throat, in particular, is a common childhood infection. The bacterium can colonize many areas of the body, including the throat, sinuses, gastrointestinal tract, anus, and urinary tract, making it necessary to investigate multiple sites if you suspect Strep but do not immediately find it with a rapid Strep test or preferably, a Strep throat culture.[40]

In children, the most common presentation of a Strep infection is Strep throat. This sore throat may begin suddenly and may be accompanied by fever, inflamed and swollen tonsils (which may also present with white patches or purulent discharge), petechiae on the hard or soft palate of the mouth, swollen lymph nodes, or other generalized symptoms like headache, abdominal pain, nausea, vomiting, and a body rash (known as scarlet fever or scarlatina). However, some children who develop PANDAS do not experience symptoms except neurobehavioral changes when exposed to close contact with Strep throat.[41]

Why PANDAS? Think Molecular Mimicry

Molecular mimicry occurs when the immune system mistakenly attacks healthy body tissues because there are structural similarities between molecules on the infectious agent and molecules on our body tissues. In rheumatic fever, this molecular mimicry can result in carditis, polyarthritis, erythema marginatum, and Sydenham's chorea.[42] In both Sydenham chorea and PANDAS, and in a genetically susceptible child, there is a misdirected immune response where the anti-Group A Strep antibodies recognize and attack the basal ganglia of the brain, causing changes to both motor function and behavior.[43]

Symptoms of PANDAS

In addition to Strep throat signs, such as pharyngeal petechiae, erythema, purulence, and swollen glands and tonsils, other signs can include strawberry tongue (raised papillae on tongue), red ring around the anus with rectal Strep, and peeling fingers or toes, usually occurring six weeks after a Strep infection, Symptoms for children with PANDAS include an acute behavioral or personality change, tics, OCD, anxiety, increased hyperactivity, behavioral regression (baby talk or only playing with significantly younger children), dysgraphia and/or somatic symptoms (urinary frequency/urgency/enuresis or sleep disturbances such as anxiety at bedtime, restless sleep, and REM disinhibition). Parents sometimes report choreiform movements ("piano-playing fingers"). Descriptions and videos of these physical findings, including the choreiform movements, can be found at www.drohara.com.

Diagnosing PANDAS

PANDAS is a **clinical diagnosis of abrupt behavioral changes** after a presumed or confirmed Strep infection.[44] No positive culture or laboratory test can make the diagnosis, and negative cultures or laboratory tests cannot deny the diagnosis. However, testing may be helpful and confirmatory and should be undertaken as below.[45]

Cultures

As mentioned previously, Strep must be thoroughly investigated and appropriately treated. Rapid Strep tests are convenient but not always reliable in finding Strep. It is recommended to culture the throat and any other tissues that may be affected, including the urinary tract and the gastrointestinal tract (rectal culture is necessary if a red anal ring is present).

Lab Markers

In examining Strep associated with PANDAS, I measure antiStreptolysin O (ASO) and antiDNaseB Ab to see if there is evidence of a recent Strep infection.[46] It may take up to eight weeks for post-infection Strep titers to appear elevated, and these antibodies only indicate that a child has had a previous Strep infection, not that the child has PANDAS.[47] In addition, a child with immunodeficiency may not mount an appropriate immune response and therefore may have negative titers. The most commonly positive test in ~ 56% of patients in our practice is a positive yet nonspecific antinuclear antibody (ANA), indicating an inflammatory or autoimmune response.[48]

To officially diagnose PANDAS, a child must be experiencing significant obsessions, compulsions, and/or tics, with an **abrupt onset** of symptoms. After the initial presentation, there may be a relapsing-remitting course of symptom severity, but the initial presentation must be acute. The neurobehavioral changes must be associated specifically with Streptococcal infection.

In atypical cases, I will sometimes perform CamKinase testing. Calcium-dependent Calmodulin Protein Kinase II is an enzyme that is involved in the upregulation of many neurotransmitters, such as dopamine.[49] The enzyme increases the sensitivity and responsiveness of neurologic receptors to neurotransmitters and is often elevated in children with PANDAS. This testing is most helpful when a child is in a flare or has significant symptoms, and the diagnosis or association with Strep or other infection is unclear.

"When CaMKII antibody-mediated activation was studied in patients with neuropsychiatric disorders such as PANDAS, TS, OCD, SC, and ADHD compared to healthy subjects, it was significantly elevated in PANDAS and acute SC (P = < 0.0001). Children diagnosed with PANDAS demonstrated antibody-mediated CaMKII enzyme activation at a mean of 150% (range = 115–198%), and those with SC had CaMKII activation of 221% (range = 194–249%) compared to normal control subjects, with a mean CaMKII activation of 93% (range = 72–112%). Sera from the children diagnosed with non-PANDAS TS, OCD, or ADHD demonstrated normal levels of CaMKII activation, despite the presence of elevated autoantibodies in some of their sera."[50]

Treatment

With throat infections, your treatment plan will change dramatically depending on throat culture results. As you know, viral infections will not be alleviated with prescription antibiotics, so it is essential to obtain a throat culture appropriately. Keep in mind that inadequately obtained Strep cultures (caused by poor patient compliance or poor technique, as previously stated) may be falsely negative. Antimicrobial treatment should be initiated if the culture is positive or Strep is likely, given the history and physical exam findings. Without effective treatment of this initial infection, Streptococcal infections can progress to scarlet fever, post-Streptococcal glomerulonephritis, rheumatic fever, and post-Streptococcal reactive arthritis. Even with effective treatment (and certainly without it), one in two hundred children may develop PANDAS.[51] Overall, early detection and treatment is of utmost importance.

Firstline therapy for Strep infection includes a round of antibiotics, typically Beta-Lactams such as Penicillin or Amoxicillin, which works well to decrease symptoms and the duration of the illness, as well as prevent the spread of Strep to others or the worsening of a child's case. Sometimes, however, a single round of antibiotics is not enough, and reculture after treatment is important. Unlike a simple Strep throat, when a child has PANDAS, the antibiotic course must be extended for three to four weeks. At times, additional antibiotics must be utilized, as mentioned in the "Considering PANDAS" chapter. With both chronic Strep infections and, of course, with PANDAS, prophylactic antibiotics must be considered. The prototype for this is the treatment and then prophylaxis of Rheumatic Fever. Refer to the chapter "Considering PANDAS" for antibiotic and antimicrobial treatment options for

PANDAS and to our membership program at www.drohara.com for more information on dosing.

MYCOPLASMA AND PANS

When a child has a history of sore throat and subsequent acute behavioral changes, *Streptococcus* should, of course, be your first focus. What if all testing comes back negative for Strep—is it still PANDAS? Perhaps not.

When the diagnostic criteria for PANDAS were introduced in the late 1990s, it excluded many children who were experiencing acute onset of neurobehavioral symptoms immediately following infection—but not with Group A Strep. Initially, other infectious causes of autoimmune encephalitis were termed PITANDS (Pediatric Infection-Triggered Autoimmune Neuropsychiatric Disorders). Understanding that Strep and other infectious agents may not be the only trigger for autoimmune encephalitis, Dr. Sue Swedo and 30 practitioners met to consolidate the diagnosis, and many agreed on the term, PANS, or Pediatric Acute-onset Neuropsychiatric Syndrome, which modified the criteria of PANDAS to include additional infectious, metabolic, and non-infectious agents. Going back to our theoretical patient with a history of acute behavioral changes but no evidence of past Strep infection, Mycoplasma should now rise to the top of your infectious differential.[52]

What is Mycoplasma?

Mycoplasma pneumoniae, an atypical bacterium, is sometimes known as "walking pneumonia," as symptoms of this infection are milder than other types of pneumonia. Much like Strep, Mycoplasma is spread through respiratory droplets, is often treatable with antibiotics, and is a fairly common culprit in children with sinusitis, bronchitis, and pneumonia.[53]

When children first present with the infection, they typically experience a low-grade fever, cough or other respiratory symptoms, fatigue, and headache, alongside possible sore throat. The symptoms may be mild and are often overlooked. Subsequently, symptoms that develop in children affected by PANS include behavioral changes, OCD, tics, anxiety, restrictive eating, and somatic symptoms, including urinary and sleep disturbances. Sometimes, as with Strep, a child may be exposed and show no evidence of physical illness at all.[54]

Diagnosing Mycoplasma

Culture-based diagnosis of Mycoplasma is not very sensitive. Blood tests usually include *Mycoplasma pneumoniae* IgG and IgM antibodies. They may not always be helpful, as antibodies can take up to 6 weeks or more to develop post-infection, may vary if the patient is immunosuppressed, and may only be reflective of a past infection unrelated to current behavioral symptoms (if only IgG is positive). Some clinicians use real-time PCR, a rapid and sensitive test that can determine acute infection, or Immunofluorescence Assay (IFA), a standard technique to identify the presence of antibodies by their ability to react with antigens expressed in cells infected with Mycoplasma.[55]

Research has demonstrated that children with chronic tic disorders (CTD) may have a propensity toward enhanced immune activation.[56] Still, Mycoplasma-induced PANS should be considered only in those with a history of ABRUPT onset of symptoms.

With the abrupt onset of neurobehavioral symptoms, titer testing for both Mycoplasma and Strep infection is appropriate. Other tests to consider, as described in previous chapters, include inflammation and autoimmunity markers such as ANA with reflex profile, ESR, and CRP, metabolic markers like MTHFR and organic acid testing, and mitochondrial function markers such as carnitine, ammonia, lactate, and total CK, as warranted.

Treating Mycoplasma

Mycoplasma is a fairly stubborn atypical bacterium. Treatment with fluoroquinolones, macrolides, or tetracyclines is appropriate, and we usually start with a macrolide such as Azithromycin or Clarithromycin.

In conjunction with prescriptive antibiotics,[57] you can consider:

- Cryptolepis, an antimicrobial and anti-inflammatory herb historically used to treat malaria[58] and now often used to treat Babesia

- Mullein is a gentle antimicrobial herb[59] with an affinity for lungs and sinus cavities.

- Colloidal silver is used orally or as a nasal spray, a natural antimicrobial that can be applied directly to the affected system (see chapter on Antimicrobials).

- Oil of oregano, elderberry (as well as other ethanol extracts)[60]

- Berberine (in the form of Goldenseal)[61]

- Houttuynia[62]

- Isatis, Chinese skullcap, curcumin, and broccoli seed extracts are also helpful in decreasing Mycoplasma-related inflammation.[63]

As discussed in the introductory chapters, our practice's three most common infections are Strep, Mycoplasma, and Bartonella. If it is not explicit from the history and physical exam as to which infectious trigger is most likely, we will often start a child on Azithromycin, given its safety profile and sensitivity to all three of these infections in our area of the country. Once test results have returned, we can then tailor a more individualized plan. Again, for more details on antibiotics and antimicrobials, see the chapter on Antimicrobials and www.drohara.com.

VIRUSES

An equally contagious trigger for PANS, viruses make up a large percentage of PANS cases, as they encompass a host of common infections like Influenza, the common cold, *Herpes simplex*, Epstein-Barr, Cytomegalovirus, and now COVID-19. With PANS and autoimmune encephalitis, viruses can be hard to identify as a trigger, as they are so ubiquitous. A detailed history of all infectious viral triggers is of utmost importance in making this diagnosis.

Diagnosing Viral-Triggered PANS

Signs and Symptoms

Common symptoms of viral infection include fever, gastrointestinal upset and/or vomiting, body rash, fatigue, nasal discharge, and respiratory symptoms. However, I must emphasize that children with PANS and PANDAS may not display any of these characteristic symptoms at all, manifesting neurobehavioral changes instead.

Classic signs of viruses include swollen and tender lymph nodes, clear discharge, and rashes, so be sure to look for these during your physical examination, as well as cold sores, aphthous ulcers, and canker sores.

Testing

Remember again that PANS is a clinical diagnosis, and testing can only be a guide. Often, chronic IgG antiviral antibodies will be positive;

a positive result only indicates past infection and is not indicative of autoimmune encephalitis. In specific circumstances, such as the abrupt onset of symptoms after a live viral vaccine, a herpes cold sore, or a mono-like illness, I will consider antiviral antibodies, including Epstein-Barr virus, Cytomegalovirus, HHV-6, and MMR or Varicella. In addition, I will review other tests, including:

- Complete blood count to determine if the infection is affecting blood cells, paying special attention to white blood cell count, neutrophils, and lymphocytes.

- Immunoglobulin panel, including IgG, IgM, IgE, and IgA with subclasses

- General signs of inflammation, especially ANA, ESR, and hs-CRP

Treatment and Ongoing Management

Conventional medicine offers relatively little when it comes to the pharmaceutical management of viral infections. However, many researchers have shown the benefits of Amantadine as an effective antiviral and anti-inflammatory, perhaps even for COVID-19.[64, 65, 66] It is a medication which has been used for decades in the treatment of Parkinson's Disease, and new research, as well as our anecdotal experience, has shown that it helps to decrease OCD and a child's tendency to "get stuck" in loops, and improves mood.[67]

Nutraceuticals can be very helpful in decreasing viral load, and we often utilize antioxidants such as Vitamins A,[68] C,[69] D,[70] and zinc,[71] which inhibit viral replication. Studies of measles and other viral encephalitides have shown that a high dose of vitamin A (in appropriate dosing and under the guidance of a practitioner) can be vital in treating the autoimmune encephalitis brought on by viruses.[72] I also often consider lysine, an amino acid that can decrease viral load, as it directly reduces arginine,[73] which promotes viral replication. Monolaurin, especially in newer forms such as Aqualaurin, which includes a biofilm buster, interferes with viral assembly and maturation[74] and may be particularly helpful if the child is in a flare from an acute viral illness.

Herbal antivirals may be helpful for both new cases of PANS and management of flares, and I turn to astragalus,[75] Andrographis,[76] berberine,[77] and elderberry.[78] These stop a virus' capability to replicate by inhibiting its ability to penetrate the cell wall. Olive leaf extract can also be helpful,[79] as it prevents viral shedding, budding, and assembly of cell membranes. Other herbal preparations I may utilize include glycyrrhizic acid (licorice)[80] which inhibits viral growth and inactivates viral particles, and lemon balm,[81] which inhibits viral replication. Unique products that are relatively new to the market but have proven very helpful include transfer factors (which decrease the production of Th17, thereby balancing immune function)[82] and specialized pro-resolving mediators (which may help to bring an overactive immune response back to balance).[83] With any abrupt onset of OCD or other neurobehavioral symptoms outlined in the PANS chapter, virally triggered autoimmune reactivity should be considered.

In addition to the viruses outlined in this chapter, we should also include COVID-19 in this list.[84] The impact of a proinflammatory immune state leading to OCD and neurobehavioral symptoms must be assessed. If COVID or other viral infection is suspected or found, antiviral, antioxidant, and anti-inflammatory treatment may mitigate not only the viral infection but also the subsequent neurobehavioral and neuropsychiatric symptoms.

Yeast Dysbiosis

Multiple studies have highlighted how gastrointestinal composition can influence behavior and brain function.[85, 86, 87] Some have investigated the relationship between PANS/PANDAS and gut microbiota ecology and have indicated that Streptococcal infections may alter gastrointestinal flora, leading to inflammation and immune response activation.[88]

Yeast may be an interesting and misunderstood "infection" in our PANS kids.[89] I use that term lightly, as yeast is a normal part of our everyday flora, and as such, yeast overgrowth is not actually an infection but an imbalance.[90] Still, an imbalanced microbiome can wreak havoc on the nervous system, so knowing the signs and symptoms of yeast overgrowth or an inability to handle an imbalance in fungal flora is important to accurately assess and appropriately manage a child in crisis.[91]

Diagnosing Yeast

The presentation of yeast overgrowth is distinctive, as a yeast-affected child's personality can appear almost drunk—he may be inappropriately silly and hyper, he could seem irrationally angry and hypersensitive, or he may appear somewhat withdrawn or lethargic. Anything that alcohol (or sugar) can do to the body, yeast can do to a child. Yeast may be hard to culture or diagnose by testing, so we need to be especially mindful of it in our history and physical exam.[92]

Common Signs and Symptoms

- Mood swings, agitation, or aggression

- Inappropriate laughter

- Thickened, ridged, yellowed, or malleable nails

- Rashes/tinea, thrush/white tongue

- Sugar or carbohydrate cravings

- Urinary frequency

- Spaciness and brain fog

Children with yeast overgrowth tend to have significant gastrointestinal involvement, experiencing gas and bloating, stinky or sweet-smelling bowel movements, resistance to weight loss, large appetites without weight gain, and sugar cravings. Sometimes we see the classic white coating on the tongue (thrush),[93] which can be quite mild and yet still indicative of yeast. Other physical findings such as dandruff or cradle cap, athlete's foot, ringworm (*Tinea capitis* or *corporis*), or other yeast rashes and nail findings are all signs of yeast overgrowth.

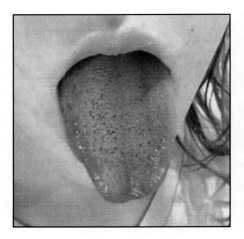

Mild Thrush/White Tongue

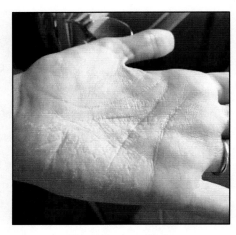

Yeast Rash on Palm

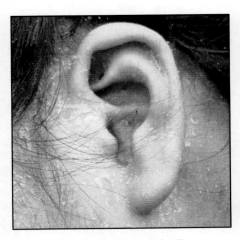

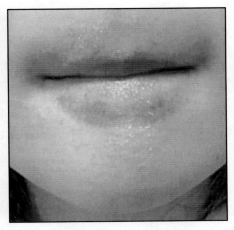

Yeast Rash Around the Ear

Fungal Infection Around the Mouth With Excessive Lip Licking

Upon physical examination, you might find a silly child with high-pitched squealing, flushed cheeks, and general sensory overload. Look for rashes, especially *Tinea capitis* or *corporis*, diaper rashes (especially in a potty-trained child), vaginal or anal irritation or inflammation, abdominal bloating, acne, or dandruff, and yellowing and thickening of the nails, and of course, thrush. In small children, nails may be malleable and just beginning to have some vertical ridges. Yeast on the skin may also fluoresce under a Wood's lamp.

Medical History

A child's medical history may be full of red flags for yeast overgrowth, including delivery by Caesarean section and infantile history of colic, reflux, thrush, diaper rash, or cradle cap. Take note of significant previous antibiotic use, constipation, diarrhea or encopresis, and sugar or carbohydrate cravings. Disturbed sleep and sudden onset of aggression and emotional volatility are also common in children affected by yeast.

Yeast is not a classic PANS infection and often does not present with an acute onset. However, both mold and yeast should be considered, especially in children with subacute or more chronic onset of symptoms and/or excessive antibiotic use. Further discussion of subacute presentations and the effects of mold, as well as Lyme, are discussed in the Chronic Inflammatory Response Syndrome (CIRS) Chapter.[94]

Tests to Consider

Investigating yeast with lab work can be difficult, and history and physical exam are truly the best biomarkers. Rarely will a stool analysis, culture, or blood Candida antibody panel (IgA, IgM, IgG) be helpful. Instead, I typically order a urine organic acid test (OAT) to investigate a host of metabolic pathways. The most accurate metabolite of yeast overgrowth is arabinitol or arabinose, though others, including tartaric acid, may be found in children with yeast overgrowth.[95, 96, 97]

Treating Yeast

I often liken treating yeast or other dysbiotic flora to fighting an enemy army. In that fight, we need to starve the enemy, in addition to bringing in the handguns and heavy artillery. That means we need to treat dysbiosis with diet, limiting sugars and simple carbohydrates, and promoting a healthy, anti-inflammatory way of eating (refer to our nutrition chapter for much more information on this). We may also need to bring in heavier artillery, like prescriptive antifungal medications (Fluconazole and Terbinafine work well).[98, 99] While using these, it is essential to monitor liver and kidney function through comprehensive metabolic panels and CBCs every two to three months to ensure no negative, unexpected, idiopathic effects. In decades of practice, I have very rarely witnessed any issues with this approach. I personally prefer systemic antifungals over Nystatin or other non-systemic medications, as the symptoms indicate a need for systemic treatment.[100]

Herbal Options

In many children, much like a steady stream of hand-to-hand combat in this analogy, I prefer using a rotation of herbal antifungals and, at times, using herbals in conjunction with or after pharmaceuticals.

My favorite herbals include:

- Oil of oregano[101]

- Grapefruit seed extract[102]

- Caprylic acid[103]

- Pau d'arco[104, 105]

- Berberine (as from goldenseal)[106]

- Plant tannins and essential oils[107]

- Allicin (as from garlic)[108]

Additional herbals, nutrients, and supplements to consider:

- Biotin: a nice adjunct to resistant yeast overgrowth[109], as insufficiency creates a hospitable environment for Candida.

- Anti-inflammatories and antioxidants such as Resveratrol[110]

- Probiotics and prebiotics, particularly containing the yeast-like strain Saccharomyces *boulardii.*[111]

If a child responds well to treatment, you should prolong it, which is when an herbal rotation can be very effective. Just as with pharmaceuticals, a child may experience a healing crisis or die-off reaction when beginning antifungal treatment. As always, start low and increase treatment intensity slowly to avoid these significant but temporary negative reactions.

Biofilm Protocol

Many children with severe or prolonged dysbiosis may require a biofilm protocol. When organisms begin to inhabit mucous membranes, they may secrete a slimy substance as a protective mechanism, which affords them shelter from antimicrobial agents.[112] This can interfere greatly with treatment, so disrupting biofilms is an important aspect of a holistic care plan. In general, biofilm protocols include:

Step 1

Lysis: break up the biofilm layer with natural, specific, or more general enzymes. Do this on an empty stomach.

Step 2

Antimicrobial: kill the germs by administering an antifungal/antimicrobial fifteen to thirty minutes after step 1. It is most beneficial to use a rotation of herbs here in order to avoid resistance.

Step 3

Mop-up: at least ninety minutes after administering the antifungal, use fiber, such as psyllium or pectin, to bind up the debris released by the dying pathogen.

Step 4

Nourish: use a wholesome diet, antioxidants, and anti-inflammatories to reduce immunologic load and support the reconstitution of the child's system.[113]

Die-Off

With any treatment of dysbiosis, but particularly with prescriptive antifungals, die-off is possible. Die-off is similar to a Herxheimer reaction, with a worsening of any of those symptoms that we are trying to decrease, including bowel or behavior changes. As such, we usually start dosing low and increase slowly to avoid these undesirable effects. However, when die-off occurs, using a binder such as activated charcoal or fiber can decrease the reaction. Keep in mind that a negative reaction is also a positive—it reminds us we are on the right track. It's the enemy army not wanting to die! It is essential to remind parents of this and to prepare ourselves for these bumps in the road.

Final Thoughts

Yeast is not commonly accepted as a PANS trigger. However, in children who have experienced excessive antibiotic use or in those who exhibit drunken or "yeasty" behaviors, treating fungal imbalance should be considered.[114]

.

Mold and Chronic Inflammatory Response Syndrome (CIRS)

Diverting from children with abrupt onset of symptoms as in PANS/PANDAS, we must consider those with a more subacute presentation. Biotoxin disease from Lyme and Lyme co-infections or mycotoxin illness from mold exposure immediately come to mind as potential sources of inflammation. With CIRS, Subtype 1, which comprises 75% of all CIRS cases, it is not just mold spore fragments that cause health disturbances but also volatile organic compounds (VOCs), microorganisms on the skin such as Actinomycetes and Mycobacteria, and the interplay with beta-glucans and proteinases, among others. As with many chronic illnesses, two factors must be kept at the top of mind: genetic susceptibility and environmental exposure. Genetic susceptibility "loads the gun," while environmental exposure merely "pulls the trigger."[115]

In cases of Chronic Inflammatory Response Syndrome or mold mycotoxin disease, a child or adolescent typically has an HLA (Human Leukocyte Antigen) genetic susceptibility and comes into contact with the mold (likely from a water-damaged building), which they are not able to detoxify appropriately. Twenty-five percent of the population is genetically prone to CIRS, and at least two percent are highly susceptible to disabling neurologic, immunologic, vascular, and endocrine symptoms when this develops. CIRS has two main types: CIRS Subtype 2, associated with Lyme Disease (which is discussed in the "Other Infections" chapter of this guidebook), and CIRS Subtype 1, associated with exposure to water-damaged buildings with Environmental Relative Moldiness Index (ERMI) scores greater than two. A staggering 75% of CIRS cases fall into the Subtype 1 category.[116]

In most people, biotoxins are either broken down by the liver or attacked and excreted by an effective immune response. However, in those with HLA susceptibility, these same biotoxins/mycotoxins that are otherwise easily excreted cause significant impairment of nerve cell function, resulting in chronic cytokine inflammatory response and leading to possible sleep disturbance, chronic pain, gastrointestinal and neurologic problems, and prolonged illness.[117]

Mold mycotoxins are ionophores, with one lipophilic end that dissolves in lipids and one hydrophilic end that dissolves in water, and are less than one micron in length. Their small size and uncanny ability to pass into and out of cells makes them easily inhaled and difficult to eradicate. People come into contact with these mold mycotoxins through inhalation, ingestion, or physical touch, and if they are not appropriately managed, a chronic inflammatory response can follow. This concept of chronic inflammation as a result of mold/mycotoxin exposure was first described by Ritchie Shoemaker, MD. He discovered improvements in biotoxin illness when fishermen were treated with binders during a Pfiesteria outbreak. His pioneering (and somewhat controversial) research on this illness and treatment are outlined well in research papers and books that he, Neil Nathan, MD, and others published.[118]

Keep in mind that mold exposure and mycotoxin illness may not be immediately considered by a family. A thorough history of symptoms as below, as well as an understanding of the patient's environment, is a vital part of the diagnosis.

Diagnosing CIRS

Symptoms of CIRS

Pathognomonic symptoms of CIRS include electric shock, lightning bolt and/or ice pick sensations, and pain.[119]

The most common signs and symptoms also include:

- Post-exertional malaise, fatigue, weakness

- Memory, concentration, executive function problems

- Headaches, vertigo, and lightheadedness

- Muscle aches, cramping, joint pains, unusual skin sensitivity

- Hypersensitivity to light, blurred vision, burning eyes

- Cough, chronic congestion, sinus, asthma-like illnesses

- Air hunger, shortness of breath

- Chronic gastrointestinal complaints, including cramping, nausea, and diarrhea

- Thirst, appetite swings, body temperature irregularities

- Urinary frequency, night sweats

- Sleep disturbances[120]

Testing

If you are considering this illness because of the presence of the symptoms listed above and suspected exposure to mold and water-damaged buildings, the first test to consider is a urine mycotoxin test.[121] This test should be done after provocation with glutathione or sweating from exercise or a sauna session to best stimulate mycotoxin release into the urine sample.[122] Another easily administered test is Visual Contrast Sensitivity (VCS), which measures neurological function through the optic nerve. Biotoxin exposure can impair optic nerves and a child's ability to see patterns. Ninety-eight percent of patients who fail a VCS test and have more than eight of the symptoms listed previously will have CIRS.[123] An MRI with NeuroQuant stratification can also be useful in identifying abnormalities related to water-damaged buildings (WDB), typically revealing increased forebrain parenchyma and cortical gray matter, as well as decreased caudate and pallidum, or as with Lyme disease, small forebrain parenchyma, putamen, and large cerebellum.[124]

Other CIRS biomarkers include:[125]

- Human leukocyte antigen (HLA-DRB and HLA-DQ) genetic susceptibility

- High C4a: excessive innate immune response to biotoxins.[126]

- High matrix metallopeptidase 9 (MMP-9): gelatinous enzyme associated with tumor invasiveness.

- Low melanocyte-stimulating hormone (MSH): a marker of neuropeptide control, suggests low production of pro-inflammatory cytokines.

- High leptin: a marker of inflammation-induced disruption of hypothalamic axis; weak correlation with CIRS

- High tumor growth factor (TGF)-beta 1: a marker of overactive, chronic immune response

- Low vascular endothelial growth factor (VEGF): a marker of capillary hypoperfusion; low endurance

- High anti-gliadin antibodies: markers of intestinal permeability and increased risk of autoimmune reactivity.

- Multiple Antibiotic Resistant Coagulase Negative Staph (MARCoNS): identified by nasal culture, indicates a barrier to immune defenses and suggests possible high colonization.[127]

Treating CIRS

The first step in treating CIRS is to remove exposure to the toxic mold, which can completely resolve all symptoms in some cases. However, this process is much easier said than done, as mold remediation is extremely challenging. Seek out mold remediation services that have experience working with health practitioners, as many mold specialists are not educated on the health impacts of mold and may not be a good match for your patients.[128]

Once remediation of the home is in place, and sometimes without remediation when it is not possible, medical treatment can begin. This should be done with a qualified and experienced clinician as warranted in each individual case. A comprehensive mold treatment will include addressing dysbiosis, using binders to decrease die-off symptoms, and supporting healthy detoxification. Although treatment will depend largely on the type of mold the child has been exposed to, the underlying genetic susceptibility, and the child's comorbidities,[129] I generally recommend:

1. Preloading with essential fatty acids, as these are neuroprotective and restorative and may work to repair the myelin sheath.

2. Treating yeast/fungal overgrowth and other dysbiosis in nasal cavities, the gastrointestinal tract, and systemically with antimicrobial herbs and/or prescriptive antifungals (see Chapter on Yeast for more details).

3. Using a binder/detoxifier such as activated charcoal or Cholestyramine to inactivate toxins released, being mindful to avoid constipation. Note that Cholestyramine may be the best binder of ochratoxins, activated charcoal for aflatoxins, and glutathione and n-acetyl cysteine for gliotoxins.

4. Use supplements to aid immune, metabolic, and detoxification support. Some of my favorite immune modulators include resveratrol, curcumin, quercetin, and CBD. Cannabinoids can also modulate glutamate, calming the nervous system.

5. Digestive aids such as enzymes, bitters, or ox bile, in combination with fiber and probiotic support, may ensure healthy bowel movements and, therefore, proper excretion of biotoxin complexes.

6. As with all chronic illness treatments, dietary interventions must be in place for optimum efficacy. Consider having patients increase the following in their diets to support normal and healthy body functions:

   a. Cruciferous vegetables, seeds, nuts, and berries are all high in antioxidants.

   b. Chicory root, artichoke leaf, and dandelion greens to stimulate natural detoxification.

   c. Spices such as curry powder, garlic, and green and black teas decrease inflammation and increase antioxidant stores.

For more information on how to support your mold-exposed patients, refer to www.drohara.com and the links below:

- www.survivingmold.com

- www.ewg.org
- www.neilnathanmd.com

Other Infections: Parasites, Clostridia, Lyme Disease, and Co-infections

Occasionally, the infectious agent responsible for PANS isn't found among the usual suspects, and we must dig a little more deeply. Though not very common, parasites and Clostridia can trigger neuroinflammation, resulting in autoimmune encephalitis. In addition, if all of the other infectious agents triggering PANS and PANDAS have been ruled out, and particularly if the onset is more subacute, Lyme and co-infections like Bartonella and Babesia, as well as mold mycotoxins (CIRS as discussed in the previous chapter), should be investigated. As previously stated, these subacute or more chronic presentations do not fit PANS and Basal Ganglia Encephalitis criteria but should be investigated in clinically significant cases.

Parasites

Parasites are an interesting category of infectious organisms because most people associate a pretty strong "ick" factor with them. Parasites are organisms that live in or on their hosts and feed off of the host's resources in order to maintain life. Despite the negative association we in an industrialized society have with parasites, they have evolved alongside the human immune system for millennia and are quite common.

There are three main categories of parasites:

- Protozoa: these must have a host to replicate, like Babesia (a Lyme co-infection).

- Helminths: these are worms, including roundworms, tapeworms, and pinworms.

- Ectoparasites: these live *on* their hosts, like lice, fleas, bedbugs, and scabies.

Again, we do not normally see parasites triggering PANS. Diagnosis for these relies mostly on a child's clinical picture. Red flag symptoms include worsening behavior around the moon cycles (especially the full moon), bruxism, itching of the buttocks and anus, and, occasionally, intense dark circles around the eyes.

Most parasites are very hard to find, but those that are sometimes positive upon testing include *Giardia lamblia*, *Dientamoeba fragilis*, and *Blastocystis hominis*. Conventional stool analysis does not often detect parasite involvement, so if using this technique, it is best to collect the stool sample around the time of a full moon and request an ova and parasites study. Several companies use DNA or PCR probe technology, which might be more helpful. On a basic CBC, elevated eosinophils could indicate parasite infection as well.[130]

Treating Parasites

With parasites, I typically prescribe pharmaceutical medications immediately, then utilize natural remedies and herbs for maintenance and flares. My go-tos include culture-proven and weight-specific doses of Metronidazole or Nitazoxanide/Alinia as well as Albendazole/Albenza, and Mebendazole/Vermox. With helminth therapy, such as HDCs, I use Praziquantel/Biltricide for infestation.[131] Although these medications are effective, we are seeing clinically that some children need longer antiparasitic treatment over the course of several weeks, so do not hesitate to extend treatment with herbal formulations if a resolution has not been satisfactory.

Among the natural remedies to consider, I recommend:

- Mimosa Pudica: an herb native to Asia whose seeds form a gel-like substance when hydrated. This not only captures GI debris and biofilms[132] it has also been shown historically to paralyze and kill parasites[133] as well. The herb has liver-protective effects and may support the repair of the GI tract.

- Artemisia spp: Several strains of artemisia are effective against parasites, and one recent study on Artemisia absinthium found that the herb may cause worm paralysis, death, and ultrastructural alterations, such as tegumental damage, lipid accumulation, and destruction of the nephridial canal and the intrauterine eggs, in a dose-dependent manner.[134]

- Juglans Nigra: More commonly known as black walnut, this herb is used as an anthelmintic and antiviral[135] so that it may be effective in children with both parasite and viral issues.

Clostridia

Clostridia is a unique subset of bacterial infection, as it is characterized by the formation of resistant endospores, making it particularly difficult to eradicate, and by the cornucopia of distinctive toxins and enzymes, it produces. These bacteria have become quite notorious throughout the centuries, causing devastating diseases such as tetanus, botulism, and gas gangrene. While modern sanitation practices have been able to reduce the frequency of these infections, Clostridia still persists.[136]

As gram-positive, distinctly anaerobic, fairly ubiquitous bacteria, Clostridia species take advantage of wounds, antibiotic use, or the ingestion of Clostridia-infested food in order to grow and release toxins. Specifically with *Clostridium difficile*, a normal constituent of a healthy microbiome, antibiotic use can devastate the gastrointestinal flora and give C. diff the opportunity it needs to become invasive and harmful. In children with a history of antibiotic use, Clostridia overgrowth is certainly a possibility and should be investigated if children show signs and symptoms of such an "infection." Clostridia species produce propionic acid, a neuroinflammatory compound that negatively impacts the central nervous system and thus can trigger neurobehavioral symptoms.[137] Though not typically considered in the differential diagnosis of PANS, if abrupt or subacute onset of neurobehavioral symptoms coincides with Clostridium signs and symptoms, then appropriate investigation and treatment should be considered.

Investigating Clostridium

When caring for children with Autism Spectrum or other neurodevelopmental disorders, pathogenic Clostridium overgrowth (of many Clostridia species, not just C. diff) may manifest as high levels of aggression, including biting, hitting, and even self-harm with head banging or repetitive motion. As mentioned previously, a child's history of antibiotic use is a key factor in assessing his risk for Clostridium overgrowth. Clostridial infection should be investigated in appropriate clinical situations, but again, it is not a typical manifestation of PANS.

Lab Markers

Stool cultures can be helpful in assessing Clostridia overgrowth, and diarrheal stools will be most positive. As with many other infectious agent investigations, I also order Organic Acid Testing (OAT). The OAT includes quantitative metabolic markers for several species of Clostridia bacteria that produce toxic compounds and alter neurotransmitter metabolism. It also includes an assessment of the inhibitory effect of Clostridia metabolites on the key enzyme dopamine beta-hydroxylase, which converts dopamine to norepinephrine. Positive OAT results for Clostridia will show high 3-(3-hydroxyphenyl)-3-hydroxypropionic acid (more commonly known as simply "HPHPA"), which is produced by C. botulinum, C. sporogenes, and C. caloritolerans, and high 4-Cresol, a marker specific to C. difficile.[138, 139]

Treating Clostridia

Prescription antibiotics are extremely helpful in managing a Clostridium infection. While Metronidazole and Vancomycin have been commonly used in the past, both have exhibited treatment failure and recurrence of infection, so drugs like Rifamycin, Fidaxomicin, and Chloramphenicol can also be considered.[140]

Botanical medicine is a good source of antimicrobial allies. A study published in 2015[141] found that Vancomycin, the drug of choice in Clostridia infection but known to lead to possible recurrence of infection, found that the combination of Vancomycin and berberine, an antimicrobial constituent found in several common herbs (like goldenseal), prevented relapse of C. diff infection. Another study in 2016[142] found that Black Seed Oil and Myrrh effectively treated active C. diff infection. In combination with herbal and pharmaceutical antimicrobials, I also focus on appropriate probiotic supplementation to restore the balance of the microbiome.[143]

...but is it Lyme?

Now that we've gone over the basics of diagnosing and managing PANS/PANDAS, I would be remiss in not mentioning Lyme as a potential trigger for subacute autoimmune encephalitis. As a physician in Connecticut (ground zero for Lyme!), the three Bs—Borrelia, Bartonella, and Babesia—are frequently among my differentials. Although the onset of Lyme is often more insidious than the abrupt onset of PANS/PANDAS, it can sometimes manifest "out of nowhere" for families. It should be considered for any child with autoimmune encephalitis, especially if that child lives in an area endemic to ticks.

Lyme disease and PANS/PANDAS are very similar in that they are both multisystem diseases that can manifest as neuropsychiatric disorders and have a waxing and waning course of healing. Unlike PANS/PANDAS, however, Lyme is often more subacute and can have an even more multisystem pathology. When considering Lyme as a trigger, we are most interested in reviewing the neuropsychiatric manifestations.

Early Lyme can be localized or disseminated (spread throughout an organ or the body). In late Lyme, 60% have joint or musculoskeletal disease, and 15% present with neuropsychiatric problems.[144] In our practice, in those with diagnosed Lyme or co-infections, seemingly 100% of the patients have neuropsychiatric symptoms–unsurprising, as we specialize in neurobehavioral health. Still, I truly believe that late/disseminated Lyme with neurologic presentation is greatly misdiagnosed, under-diagnosed, and under-appreciated.

Diagnosing Lyme

There are dozens of species of Borrelia, which can all be transmitted via hard-body ticks of the genus *Ixodes*. These ticks have a variety of hosts, including mice, rats, shrews, squirrels, domesticated animals, and lizards. Humans can also become incidental hosts of Lyme and may transmit the infection gestationally.[145]

We used to say that if a tick was attached for less than 24 hours, it was not a problem. Now, we know better. Although there is no guaranteed minimum time of transmission, it follows that the longer the tick is attached, the higher the transmission rate. The Borrelia spirochete or any of the other Lyme co-infections can well be transmitted within the first 24 hours, and by 60 hours post-bite, that transmission risk rises to at least fifty percent. One of our newer Borrelia species, *Borrelia miyamotoi*, does not need to be fully engorged to transmit, making it one of the most infectious strains yet.[146, 147]

The International Lyme and Associated Diseases Society (ILADS) makes recommendations on testing and treatment of Lyme. When evaluating for Lyme, standard Lyme serology may play a minimal role, as negative results are highly likely. We may attribute this "false negative" finding to insufficient time between infection and testing or the patient's inability to mount an appropriate antibody response.[148]

The testing of the tick itself is optional but does not delay prophylaxis. I hear a lot of parents say, "Oh, we had to wait until the tick came back. It's positive, so now we'll treat it." This delay makes a severe course of the disease more likely. I encourage all of my families to consider treating tick bites immediately to give them the greatest chance of a swift recovery.

Signs and Symptoms of Acute Lyme Disease

Previous teachings on Lyme insisted that if a bullseye rash did not appear, it was not Lyme disease. Updated research has actually shown that 20-30% of adults, and in our practice, up to 80% of children, will not develop a noticeable post-bite rash at all, so don't wait for the rash to appear! Pay attention to other symptoms, most especially summer flu, headache, fatigue, stiff neck, muscle aches, paresthesia (numbness and tingling), sore throat, and malaise.[149]

The Rash

There is a dermatological rash typical of Lyme disease called the "EM rash"—Erythema migrans. It is a central clearing with a raised expanding border and is usually oval but can be circular. It's typically red, sometimes faint, or almost purple. It can also be solid throughout without rings, appearing as a solid circle. It is often hard to find when it's in the skin folds or hairy areas. It can spread, and it is usually painless and warm. It can be itchy, and you can usually feel it. Please refer to the photos below, as well as further presentations and information at www.drohara.com.

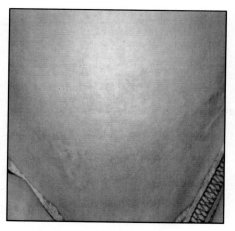

Erythema Migrans Day 1
(more bruised look in the groin)

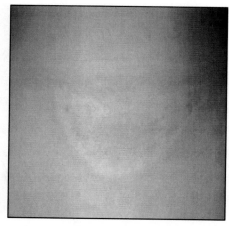

Erythema Migrans Day 2
(somewhat more classic
appearance)

Treatment

The best treatment of a disease is, of course, prevention! Most people are unaware that they have been bitten by a tick, as they are usually painless. I urge patients and practitioners alike to know the endemic areas and assume ticks are there. Take necessary precautions to reduce the possibility of a bite, including tucking in pants, wearing long sleeves and hats, and performing routine tick checks daily and after spending time outdoors. I do not personally use or encourage the use of DEET to repel ticks because of how chemically sensitive our children tend to be. However, I feel that many of the natural tick repellent formulas work well.

Treatment Basics

There is a lot to say about treating suspected Lyme, so I'll start by clarifying which treatments are typically ineffective.

There are some studies using single-dose Doxycycline with some success, but we're finding that a single dose may miss early disease, especially if there is no Erythema migrans rash. In fact, the efficacy of single-dose Doxycycline is only 50%, and it may lead to seronegative disease later. Fearing over prescription and antibiotic resistance, many primary care doctors choose to observe symptoms for six weeks and treat later, but this may actually exacerbate the late disease. Topical, long-acting, or multi-dose treatment that is less than 21 days in duration fails to show efficacy in human trials.[150]

The initial treatment ranges from three to six weeks, with Doxycycline as the preferred agent. However, giving Doxycycline in the summertime can be fraught with issues. We want parents and their children to be outside, and we want everyone to play in the dirt, but Doxycycline can cause a severe red rash all over the body when patients are exposed to the sun. When children on Doxycycline are outside, ensure they wear a big floppy hat and a rash guard. In older children, you can consider using Minocycline instead, thereby minimizing the side effect of photosensitivity. If a child is too young for either of those, you may use Amoxicillin, and if they have an Amoxicillin allergy, use a Cephalosporin or Azithromycin.[151]

Ongoing assessments are critical, especially if symptoms persist or if they progress, and education plays a large role in this. Be sure to advise parents and caregivers about additional needs and consequences of long-term antibiotic use, such as probiotics to restore balanced flora, nutrients, and herbs to protect and heal gastrointestinal cells, natural ways to reduce systemic inflammation, and prevent additional tick bites, and potential antibiotic resistance. It is common for a Herxheimer reaction to occur as you start treatment, so be sure to arm caregivers with knowledge about what this may look like and how to decrease the severity of it (binding agents work well here). If there has been an extended family history of Lyme disease or symptoms persist after an initial round of treatment, you may need an extended course of care. Other herbals and biofilm disruptors should be considered.[152]

Herxheimer Reaction

In naturopathic and homeopathic philosophies, patients often experience what's called a "healing crisis" when the correct treatment is prescribed—essentially, it'll get a little bit worse before it gets better. What we know in infectious disease as a "Herxheimer reaction" is much the same. A classic Herxheimer reaction happens as endotoxin-like products are released by harmful microorganisms as they begin to die off, especially at the onset of antimicrobial therapy. "Herxing" is actually a great sign that the antibiotic is working effectively, though not a pleasant thing for children to experience just as they are beginning their journeys with you. Eliciting this healing crisis but arming parents with ways to ease the discomfort will be vital in maintaining your patients' trust and confidence.[153]

Additional products that may help are known under the umbrella of "binders." Any natural substance that binds up these endotoxins can be incredibly useful, and our first choice is almost always activated charcoal. Other considerations may include zeolite, chlorella, diatomaceous earth, and pectin. A prescription we sometimes use is Cholestyramine, which binds fat toxins and is useful for many other inflammatory conditions. Using it initially for mold/mycotoxins and then for Lyme, Dr. Ritchie Shoemaker has been a pioneer in the effective treatment of these conditions. I would recommend learning his protocols if you are interested in this particular perspective.[154]

Research notes that Herxheimer reactions can happen in about 20% of children. Still, clinically, we have seen it much more frequently than that, especially if children start with a full dose of natural or prescription antibiotics. Note that herxing can begin within hours of treatment and can last up to a couple of weeks if not addressed appropriately.

Use the Herxheimer reaction to help inform your treatment plan. If you are not seeing symptoms resolving in the first few days or there was no Herxheimer reaction and no improvement, you may need to switch the antibiotic/antimicrobial. Continue to look for other diagnoses, as the culprit may not be *Borrelia burgdorferi* but one of the other tick-borne diseases or a different co-infection.

Treatment Failure

As with any disease, certain factors can help us determine a child's risk of treatment failure. Research and my own clinical experience have shown that treatment is difficult if the child presents with multiple rashes or multiple symptoms, if there is neurologic involvement if the child has been chronically ill before starting therapy, if initially there is no response or an incomplete response, or if there are multiple co-infections.[155] In many cases, however, the use of herbal remedies improves outcomes.[156]

Speaking of Co-Infections

Many ticks endemic to our area contain Borrelia, Bartonella, and Babesia species.[157] The two most common co-infections we encounter with neuropsychiatric effects are Bartonella and Babesia, both of which can include the symptoms of anxiety and agitation.[158] Tics and OCD are often common with Bartonella. Other signs and symptoms include striae (blanching and not along dermal lines) and other rashes, sole and heel pain, tics, tremors, fatigue, and cognitive impairments.[159]

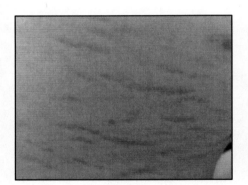 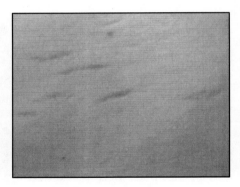

Classic Bartonella Striae on the Backs of Two Different Children

Babesia symptoms include paresthesia, head pressure, rib pain, night sweats, and air hunger. Misophonia is a common complaint as well.[160]

Diagnosing Lyme Disease

When we evaluate a child, determining the correct diagnosis can be extremely tricky, and we may consider ordering specialty labs.

Unfortunately, specialty labs are extremely cost-prohibitive, and many of our families cannot afford them. This is why I approach Lyme as a clinical diagnosis supported by test results rather than a diagnosable disease through lab values alone.

In addition to the limited accessibility of Lyme testing in the first place, completed blood work may not be positive for several weeks. You may need to look at an extended Western blot, as typical laboratories only perform a very rudimentary Western blot. PCR may have poor sensitivity. These tests can also miss co-infections, and you may also need to consider co-infection testing and treatment, especially for Bartonella and Babesia, as listed above. Some clinicians use CD57 testing, but the bottom line with Lyme testing is that it is not fully sensitive. There are a lot of false negatives, and unfortunately, finding a very normal CD57 does not rule out the disease at all.[161]

Lab Markers

So what should we look for in lab tests? The most important biomarkers, as always, are history and physical exam.[162] General inflammatory markers might be very helpful. If a child has evidence of inflammation, it should automatically trigger an investigation into autoimmune or inflammatory conditions and diseases.[163] Rule out other infections such as Strep, Mycoplasma, or viruses.

Metabolic markers may also be helpful because many of these levels are abnormal in children with Lyme disease.[164] Pay special attention to zinc, magnesium, thyroid markers, and glutathione. Investigate vitamin B12 levels, which should be measured via an MMA, methylmalonic acid. Testing a B12 level in the blood only looks at serum B12 levels, not intracellular ones, but MMA can give us a more complete picture. A high

MMA indicates your child may have a low intracellular B12 level, which can be the culprit of some neurological symptoms.

Mitochondria are the most sensitive parts of all of our cells. When there is an infection of any sort, the mitochondria are often the first to take a hit, resulting in less energy and stamina. Our children may appear tired with low tone and constipation, or they could be abnormally revved. A child with Lyme disease is susceptible to other germs, so look for other additional sources of infection, too. Consider testing for mold-related illness and Chronic Inflammatory Response Syndrome (CIRS) by ordering a urine mycotoxin test.

Some practitioners are tempted to go deeper into MRI neuro quants and SPECT scans. Still, these may be unnecessarily invasive and very expensive and are unlikely to be covered by insurance. I truly believe we need to help parents navigate the overwhelming financial impact of chronic illness, so avoiding unnecessary diagnostics and prioritizing high-quality treatment instead is paramount.

When a child presents with more subacute symptoms, I will consider and dig deeper for evidence of a previous infection-triggered abrupt onset scenario, as well as evidence of CIRS with either mold and mycotoxin disease or Borrelia, Bartonella, and/or Babesia. If a child presents with more subacute or chronic Lyme or Lyme co-infection symptoms, the interventions must address the multisystem nature of this disease. They may also include comprehensive herbal interventions, such as Japanese knotweed and other herbs.[165] The discussion of this and its multifaceted treatment is beyond the scope of this guidebook but will be discussed in more detail in our membership and mentoring program. Find out more at www.drohara.com.

STEP 1: ERADICATE THE PATHOGEN

All About Antimicrobials

Note: further guidance on treatment, including dosages and preferred brands, is available through membership and mentorship options at www.drohara.com

'

ALL ABOUT ANTIMICROBIALS

I talk about the "three-pronged approach" of antimicrobials, anti-inflammatories, and symptom management quite a bit when it comes to PANS/PANDAS because it truly is the most effective and research-proven approach to successfully managing this disease.[166] Once we have established that PANS/PANDAS or Basal Ganglia Encephalitis is at play, equally important to the success of treatment is identifying the correct infectious or triggering agents and finding an ideal combination of antimicrobials to combat them.

In general, initial antimicrobial treatment for a child with PANS/PANDAS lasts at least three to four weeks. If the agent successfully diminishes symptoms within that time, consider longer-term antimicrobials and prophylactic dosing to prevent second or third iterations of this disorder, as these often lead to more severe neuropsychological exacerbations.[167] Consider a few antibiotic and antimicrobial intervention trials if initial treatment is unsuccessful. It is also important to reevaluate the underlying infectious trigger if initial treatment is not helpful.

Determining which antibiotic to start with can be a process, but here are some considerations I like to keep in mind:

- Which germs are most likely involved, based on history and physical exam (whether or not these are confirmed by laboratory testing)?

- Previous antibiotics/antimicrobials use (for example, a child who has had multiple rounds of Amoxicillin may not respond to further penicillins).

- Local area resistance (for example, some areas have greater resistance to Azithromycin and other macrolides in the treatment of Strep or Mycoplasma)

Although I am an advocate for the frequent and regular use of herbal antimicrobials, in the early treatment of PANS/PANDAS, it is often best to use prescriptive antibiotics first. There is a tremendous amount of evidence for the use of these antibiotics in the specific treatment of PANS/PANDAS, and the positive effects in reversing symptoms are often more rapid than with herbal formulas. It is critical that we address PANS/PANDAS aggressively when it presents, then modify the long-term plan to include integrative therapies once symptoms have calmed.[168]

Laboratory Workup

If a Strep throat culture is positive, a follow-up culture should be performed after finishing antibiotic treatment. Retreatment is recommended if the culture remains positive. If a child responds poorly to two to three courses of antibiotics or continues to have frequent exacerbations despite the confirmed diagnosis, family members should be examined for Strep and Mycoplasma, as they may be a source of constant reinfection. If any are positive, treat the contact with antibiotics and retest as necessary.

Remember that PANS and PANDAS are clinical diagnoses, confirmed or not by laboratory evidence. Do not use titers to prove the diagnosis, only to help confirm it. See previous chapters on PANS and PANDAS for a complete guide to laboratory work up.

Initial Antibiotic Therapy

Because of its immune modulation, decreased incidence of negative GI symptoms, and ability to address coexisting Mycoplasma (frequently found alongside Strep), we often start antibiotic therapy with a macrolide like Azithromycin.[169] Macrolides inhibit bacterial protein synthesis, and although there are reports of macrolide-resistant Group A Streptococcus, the benefits of this class of drugs extend beyond its antimicrobial action. These drugs alter cytokine balance, downregulating NF-kB signaling and promoting apoptosis of inflammatory cells, which make them excellent anti-inflammatory agents as well.[170] Although safe for long-term use, if an initial round of Azithromycin is effective in decreasing symptoms and treatment is continued long term, ensure that an EKG is obtained to rule out a prolonged QT interval (a rare but documented effect in adults with the use of macrolides).[171]

In addition to macrolides, beta-lactam antibiotics like penicillins and cephalosporins are excellent frontline antibiotics to consider.[172] These drugs demonstrate a neuroprotective role in vitro and in vivo, and they promote the expression of the glutamate transporter, GLT1. The combination of Amoxicillin and Clavulanate (Augmentin) can be additionally effective, as clavulanic acid is anti-inflammatory and anxiolytic. Cefdinir and other cephalosporins have also shown significant improvements in tics and OCD in clinical trials over placebo.

Tetracyclines are not typically prescribed to children with PANS/PANDAS, as they have limited effects against Group A Streptococcus. However, current evidence shows that this class of drugs has substantial immunomodulatory effects[173] and can therefore be considered for this therapeutic action. Of note, tetracyclines have proven helpful against Mycoplasma, Borrelia, and Bartonella, and they can reduce oxidative stress. Still, there are side effects to consider, including sunburn-like rashes following sun exposure caused by Doxycycline, tooth discoloration, and, rarely, pseudotumor cerebri associated with Minocycline use.[174] Given these risks, these antibiotics should only be considered in children eight years and older and discussed in detail with families before they are prescribed. With all antibiotics, but especially the use of these broad-spectrum agents, the addition of probiotics and ensuring overall gut health is imperative. Make sure that the child is stooling and has gastrointestinal supportive measures in place. Please review our central hub at www.drohara.com for more information on probiotics and gut health.

In addition, it is important to remember that the GI tract begins in the nose and mouth, so appropriate treatment of gut dysbiosis or germ overgrowth begins with an oral probiotic. A study by Di Pierro et al. demonstrated that the "prophylactic administration of S. salivarius K12 to children with a history of recurrent oral Streptococcal disease resulted in a considerable reduction of episodes of both Streptococcal and viral infections, and reduced the number of days under antibiotic and/or antipyretic therapy and days of absence from school or work."[175] Although individual children may react negatively to some probiotics, *Streptococcus thermophilus*, commonly found in broad-spectrum probiotics, is safe and associated with various health benefits. Strep thermophilous is the same genus as GABHS but lacks the pathogenic M protein (STM6P); it does not induce Strep antibodies.

Finally and importantly, even if you can not determine the exact infectious trigger, JCAP guidelines recommend an extended course of antibiotics to treat Strep. We also recommend this for those with identified Mycoplasma as well as other infectious triggers such as Borrelia, Babesia, and Bartonella, as outlined in those chapters.

Long-Term Antimicrobial Treatment

After the initial use of prescription antibiotics, we will often wean them to prophylactic dosages and/or replace them with antimicrobial herbs. Below are some of the more common herbs we consider (though others may also be considered), grouped by infectious agents.

Streptococcus

- *Usnea Barbata*: commonly called "Old Man's Beard," a lichen high in usnic acid, which has demonstrated inhibition of growth of multi-resistant strains of *Streptococcus aureus,*[176] Enterococci,[177] and Mycobacteria.

- *Eleutherococcus Senticosus*: also known as "Siberian Ginseng" or Taiga, a pine needle extract with antimicrobial[178] and antifungal activity, in addition to its immunomodulatory and antioxidative properties

- *Hydrastis Canadensis* (Goldenseal) or *Berberis vulgaris* (barberry): both are high in berberine sulfate, which blocks the adherence of Streptococcus to epithelial cells and fibronectin.[179]

- *Azadirachta Indica:* commonly known as neem, is effective against several Strep species[180] responsible for dental caries.[181]

- *Origanum Vulgare*: oregano has shown high antimicrobial activity against resistant species of Streptococcus.[182]

- *Colloidal Silver*: kills five different strains of Strep and is effective against Mycoplasma and fungal infections as well.[183]

- *Cordyceps Sinensis*: medicinal mushroom-like fungus which has proven protective and immunomodulating effects against several different microbes.[184]

- *Allium Sativum*: garlic is effective against many microbial species.[185]

Mycoplasma

- *Berberine*: administered in the form of goldenseal or Oregon grape, as above.

- *Houttuynia Cordata*: a potent antiviral herb that is also effective against Mycoplasma.[186]

- Also, consider isatis, pomegranate, olive oil, reishi mushrooms, thyme, and oregano, or combination formulations available from a multitude of well-researched sources and discussed in the chapter on Mycoplasma.

Viruses

- Antioxidants such as Vitamin A, D, and zinc inhibit viral replication.[187]

- *N-acetyl-L-cysteine (NAC):* inhibits viral replication and inflammation.[188]

- *Lysine*: an essential amino acid that can decrease viral load[189]

- *Monolaurin*: a chemical made from lauric acid and commonly found in coconut oil and breastmilk, interferes with virus assembly and viral maturation. Do not use it if the child has a coconut allergy.[190]

- *Sambucus Nigra*: more commonly known as elderberry, contains hemagglutinin protein and has been shown to stop a virus' capability to replicate by inhibiting its ability to penetrate the cell wall; raw elderberries should not be consumed as they contain cyanogenic glycosides and must be cooked sufficiently to avoid the risk of cyanide toxicity.[191]

- *Glycyrrhiza Glabra*: better known as licorice, is high in glycyrrhizic acid, which inhibits virus growth and inactivates virus particles.[192]

- *Olea Europaea*: olive leaf extract prevents virus shedding, budding, and assembly of cell membranes.[193]

- *Melissa officinalis*: lemon balm can be calming and inhibits viral replication.[194]

- *Echinacea Purpurea*: increases antibody production and increases and stimulates the activity of white blood cells but should only be used for short-term therapy (less than two weeks).[195]

Yeast

- Grapefruit seed extract: inhibits *Candida albicans* biofilm development.[196]

- Berberine in the form of goldenseal as above

- Oil of Oregano: high in two potent antifungal constituents, thymol and carvacrol, which halt or inhibit the growth of *Candida albicans*.[197]

- Pau d'Arco: Candida inhibitor is especially helpful if the child also has mold toxicity.[198]

- *Gymnema Sylvestre*: blocks the virulence properties of *Candida albicans* and provides beneficial effects in treating polyphagia, fatigue, blood glucose, and lipid profile abnormalities.[199, 200]

- Caprylic acid as a stand-alone or as found in Coconut/MCT oil.[201]

- Multitude of additional combination herbal formulas may be considered.

Parasites

- *Artemisia Annua*: sweet wormwood, a bitter herb that can eliminate multiple parasites, including tapeworms and those associated with malaria and schistosomiasis.[202]

- *Juglans Nigra*: black walnut is used to expel various worms and parasites that live in the gastrointestinal tract.[203]

- *Mimosa Pudica*: gelatinous-like herb (when exposed to water) that inactivates the larvae of parasitic worms.[204]

- Coconut oil/MCT oil (as above).

- *Cucurbita Pepo*: pumpkin seeds, high in cucurbitine, fatty acids, and the protoberberine alkaloids berberine and palmatine are anthelmintic, preventing egg hatching and inhibiting worm motility.[205]

STEP 2:
IMMUNOTHERAPY

HDCs: Helminth Therapy

Inflammation

The Addition of Antioxidants

Nutrition

Note: further guidance on treatment, including dosages and preferred brands, is available through membership and mentorship options at www.drohara.com

HDCs: Helminth Therapy

I have been working with children with neurobehavioral disorders since 1988, first as a teacher and then as a physician. I have gotten to know some remarkable clinicians and scientists along the way. One of these brilliant minds is Dr. Sidney Baker.

I began working with Dr. Baker in 1997, learning, absorbing, and beginning to utilize his wisdom in treating children with a wide array of neurodevelopmental disorders.

A few "Sidisms," as we call them, include:

- "Have we done enough for this child?"

- "If you listen, they will come."

- "If you are sitting on two tacks and remove one, you do not feel 50% better."

- "We care for the child, not the disease."

- "Follow those who seek the truth and flee from those who found it." —Vaclav Havel

One of the interventions that Sid researched and considered was helminth therapy. Way back when, roundworms were used as an experimental therapy for many autoimmune disorders, and while it had its challenges, the basic premise of this therapy was extremely promising. Since then, "helminthic therapy" has evolved into a less risky, more affordable, and simpler technique that can be an incredibly powerful tool in treating patients with autoimmune disorders.[206]

Autoimmune diseases such as PANS/PANDAS and Basal Ganglia Encephalitis are a relatively new development, as they have only become prevalent since the industrialization of our world. Because preindustrial societies did not experience the plethora of autoimmune issues we see today, it follows that these diseases are not solely genetic but also have environmental triggers. These environmental factors have been identified in a multitude of studies. They include: vitamin D deficiencies related to decreased exposure to the outdoors,[207] chronic and ongoing stresses, replacement of breast milk with infant formula,[208] and an increase in Cesarean section births,[209, 210] antibiotic and antibacterial soap use,[211] shoes, toilets, and all factors that lead to a decrease in the diversity of our human biome.[212]

This depletion of and reduced diversity in the modern human biome plays a key role in the development of disease states. As we know, at least 43% of children now experience at least one chronic illness. A very readable treatise, *Epidemic of Absence,*[213] and a myriad of scientific journal articles discuss the impact of this missing microbiota on chronic inflammation, subsequent destabilizing of the immune system, and devastating neurodevelopmental issues that may ensue.[214] Through this research, it has become clear that pharmaceutical interventions are only one part of the "name it, blame it, tame it" medicine model that may no longer suffice to adequately treat disease. What is essential to the prevention and treatment of chronic diseases is the normalization and rebalancing of the gut and the immune system, promoting immune tolerance.[215]

A Balancing Act

Scientists postulated that parasites could play a part in this normalization. Still, decades of research have proven that the safe isolation and use of many nematodes, including roundworms, is expensive and problematic. It was vital to reestablishing a healthy microbiome with organisms that posed less risk to their human hosts while positively impacting neuroinflammatory conditions. Helminths emerged as a leading choice.[216]

Helminths, or worms that live in the intestines of all mammals, are mutualist organisms in the form of microscopic eggs, interacting with their host to both parties' benefit. This differs greatly from the actions of a parasite, as parasitic interactions occur when one organism (the parasite) benefits and the host is harmed.

The larval stage of the helminth has proven most therapeutically beneficial. *Hymenolepis diminuta cysticercoids*, grown in grain beetles, were commonly in our food supply up until about 100 years ago. They are now emerging as a safe and inexpensive choice for replenishing our microbiomes and recalibrating our immune systems, causing little to no adverse reactions and retraining the host immune system. Thus, HDCs provide the following advantages:

- Low cost to cultivate

- No human-to-human transmission

- Easily ingested orally (every 2-3 weeks), in a similar manner to probiotics.

- Intraluminal colonization, so no risk of infection and minimal risk of infestation (1/1000 in children).

- Raised in grain beetles, which are normally found in the human food supply—all potential contaminants in the cultivation and isolation of HDCs are already consumed by humans and are therefore safe.

It should be noted that HDCs are one life stage of *Hymenolepis diminuta* meant to normalize the immune system naturally, so although HDCs are not *the* answer for biome reconstitution, they can be a part of it. There will be variability in their effects, and they are not a quick fix, often taking up to six months to see improvements. Other medications, vitamins, minerals, probiotics, and nutraceuticals are needed to assist in any compromised system, but HDCs should be a consideration when caring for children and adults with autoimmune diseases.

Diversity and Tolerance for a Happier Biome

Tolerance is the treasure trove of all complex systems, whether they be social, political, mechanical, or physiologic; diversity is its partner. As organisms in our human biome have become less diverse, we have become less tolerant, leading to the rise in autoimmune disease, allergy, and atopy. Encouraging diversity and tolerance in the human biome is a crucial piece of the autoimmune puzzle.[217]

Primobiotics™ is one brand of HDCs that promotes tolerance in a diverse biome. As such, they are not meant to treat any specific disease, but much like probiotics can be a foundational treatment. They are a consideration for an individual with chronic illness, as they are inexpensive and safe when utilized under the care of a knowledgeable practitioner.[218]

Taking the First Steps

Some individuals are very sensitive to both immune (pollens, allergens, foods, molds, chemicals) and sensory (touch, sound, light, smell, taste) stimuli. These individuals will need to utilize a lower dose of HDCs, or they may show indications that a dose is inciting a healing crisis. These healing crises can include insomnia, hyperactivity, or digestive discomfort. Others may need a higher dose, increased gradually, to see any positive effect. HDCs are remarkably hardy and are not bothered by antifungals or antibiotics, but medications aimed specifically at worms and some probiotics containing *Lactobacillus* can decrease their effectiveness.

There are a few things to consider before utilizing HDCs.[219] First, stools must be regular and healthy. Slow transit time (longer than normal for a beet or charcoal capsule to pass) or frank constipation should be treated first. Individuals, especially children, on immunocompromising medications should seek the advice of a qualified practitioner first and should avoid HDCs. Finally, nonverbal children with autism and preexisting abdominal pain cannot readily communicate an increase in negative symptoms, so these children should be monitored regularly if they are put on this treatment at all.

Any infestation can be treated with one day of prescription Biltricide. Still, such infestation and discomfort should be avoided by following the above guidelines, working with an experienced practitioner, and using extreme caution in young, constipated, immunocompromised, or nonverbal children. Beyond these considered limitations, helminth therapy can be an excellent adjunct in immunomodulatory support of children and adults with autoimmune diseases.[220]

Dr. Baker's use and understanding of Primobiotics™ has been one of his many gifts to me and to many other practitioners. His guidance, mentorship, and love are with me daily and with every child.

INFLAMMATION

By now, you're probably familiar with the concept of inflammation, which is a natural process through which the body protects itself from damage caused by illness, injury, toxins, and other irritants. By and large, inflammation is a beneficial process, as it protects otherwise healthy tissue from damage and calls our attention to an area that needs tending. The problem arises when inflammation goes unchecked, is persistent, or attacks self (as in autoimmune disorders). Inflammation and immunological factors are increasingly recognized as vital to the discussion of neuropsychiatric disorders.[221]

Investigating Inflammation

How do you know if a child is in an (unhealthy) inflammatory state? Sometimes, it isn't so easy to tell. Inflammation can look like fatigue, sluggishness, body aches, headaches, sadness, or constipation. However, it can also look like hyperactivity, irritability, anxiety, or diarrhea. People often do not know that low-grade inflammation affects their child, so we look to simple blood tests for more insight. Elevations of erythrocyte sedimentation rate, C-reactive protein, antinuclear antibodies, and/or acute phase reactants (such as platelets and ferritin levels) can be key findings in those with chronic inflammation. The implications of elevations in antineuronal antibodies in movement disorders, including autoimmune encephalitis of many sorts, have been researched for decades.[222, 223, 224, 225, 226, 227]

I like to check a child's CBC for many reasons, including platelets, elevated as an acute phase reactant, and eosinophils. Elevated eosinophils, of course, indicate an allergic response but can also suggest the presence of parasites, a very infrequent culprit in a PANS picture, but an infection we would want to eliminate all the same.[228] Just more food for thought.

Histamine and Inflammation

Another long-known, often discussed, and more recent hot topic is mast cells. Mast Cell Activation Syndrome (MCAS)/Mast Cell Mediator Disorders (MCMD) have been implicated in many allergic, gastrointestinal, and immune-related diseases.[229] Mast cells can indeed play a role in allergies, clearance of pathogens, visceral hypersensitivity, and most recently, COVID-19.[230] Although tryptase is frequently used for diagnosis, it is often not secreted, and the timing of measurement, based on patient symptoms and the circadian clock, can be difficult. Symptoms include "pruritus, flushing, syncope, gastric distress, nausea and vomiting, diarrhea, bone pain, and neuropsychiatric symptoms, most of which are controlled by medication."[231] As of this writing, there is no cure for MCMDs, so intervention should be based on preventing mast cell stimulation, as well as reduction of effects in a slow and stepwise approach, as is indicated in most inflammatory conditions. Though further discussion of MCMDs is beyond the scope of this guidebook (but is discussed further in our mentoring program), below are listed several interventions to consider in children with PANS/PANDAS and/or when MCMD is implicated:[232]

- Antihistamines (Cetirizine, Diphenhydramine, Hydroxyzine)

- Antihistamines with anti-eosinophilic action (Ketotifen)

- Antihistamines with anti-serotonin action (Cyproheptadine)

- Tricyclic antidepressants with combined antihistamine action (Doxepin)

- Flavonoids (luteolin, quercetin of high purity)

- Antileukotrienes (Montelukast)

- Cromolyn sodium

- Steroids (Methylprednisolone)

- Epinephrine (EpiPen, AnaPen)

- Anti-IgE (Omalizumab)[233]

Inflammation Is Found. Now What?

Many interventions are used to treat inflammation. Diet is probably the most important, as it sets a foundation for all other treatments (see Nutrition chapter for more on this). A successful PANS/PANDAS protocol will not only incorporate antibiotics or antimicrobials but will also include anti-inflammatories (natural and/or pharmaceutical) and antioxidants to reduce cellular stress.[234] More often than not, addressing and managing inflammation caused by infection, metabolic imbalance, or other immunologic factors is key to effectively managing neurobehavioral and mental health.[235]

Food as Medicine

When we first interview a family, we examine the child's diet. We look to ensure it is as "anti-inflammatory" as possible.[236] Ideally, a child's diet should include food in its "whole" form, as organic and non-processed as possible. Foods high in antioxidants, such as berries, artichokes, kale, spinach, beets, dandelion greens, and red cabbage, are essential.

When it comes to sweets, dark chocolate is perfect, though admittedly a harder sell for young children. Items sweetened with honey (for children over one year), monk fruit, dates, and pure maple syrup can be a delicious addition to the diet and depending on the child's palate, a stevia leaf is also a great option. In fact, whole-leaf stevia has been shown to act as a natural Borrelia inhibitor[237] and, therefore, may be a great adjunct for children battling Lyme disease. This herb is also well known to provide a multitude of antioxidant benefits.[238]

Increasing filtered water intake, which is admittedly easier said than done, can be very impactful, especially in our children with chronic illness and dysautonomia.[239, 240] My rule of thumb for water intake is one cup (8 ounces) for every year of life, up to about 80-85 ounces after the age of 8. Sodas and other sugary beverages count against that total, so encourage limiting, if not completely eliminating, those with the family if possible. If a child suffers from POTS (Postural Orthostatic Tachycardia Syndrome) or Dysautonomia, higher amounts of water, flavored water, and salt may be essential.

Herbs and spices—particularly garlic, ginger, oregano, and turmeric—add flavor and health benefits to anything and everything. Use these with vegetable chips or homemade popcorn as added sprinkles to boost an otherwise neutral snack. Encouraging families to season eggs, oatmeal, and avocado toast with these makes a power-packed breakfast.

Healthy oils are also important, and my favorites include extra virgin olive, avocado, and coconut oils. Coconut oil is a great investment, as it is also a natural antimicrobial and source of caprylic acid. Meats should be grass-fed organic or wild-caught fish. Vegetables should be organic and local, if possible. Remove additives, sugars, gluten, casein, soy, and any food sensitivities as much as possible and as warranted. Please refer to the guidebook's Nutrition chapter or mentoring program at www.drohara.com for much more guidance.

Anti-Inflammatory Interventions

- Essential Fatty Acids (EFAs): Omega 3 (EPA/DHA) and 6 (GLA)[241]

- SPMs (specialized pro-resolving mediators)[242]

- Aloe[243]

- Curcumin[244]

- Flavonoids: quercetin, luteolin, rutin[245]

- CBD Oil[246]

- Gabapentin

- Amantadine (see Chapter on Viruses)

As previously mentioned, anti-inflammatories are key components of a successful treatment plan for many chronic diseases, especially for PANS/PANDAS. Essential fatty acids are a great foundational intervention, although you might be more familiar with them as Omega-3s, particularly EPA and DHA, or Omega 6, GLA.[247, 248] These are readily available over the counter or through a healthcare practitioner. To be honest, I find that children—humans in general—do not consume enough EFAs through diet alone. Still, it is important to eat your medicine as much as possible, and a very good food source of EFAs is sardines. It can be hard to get children to eat sardines, and let's face it; most adults don't really love sardines either. But you can consider sneaking some into pizza, salad dressing, or spaghetti! Research shows that EFAs modulate different inflammatory reactions, lowering triglycerides and improving nerve transmission. "Nerve transmission" is how cells communicate with each other and are essential to brain health and detoxification.[249, 250]

Specialized Pro-Resolving Mediators

An anti-inflammatory measure that isn't necessarily well-known is specialized pro-resolving mediators or SPMs. SPMs are derived from essential fatty acids and have important roles in orchestrating the resolution of tissue inflammation, or "catabasis." Pro-resolving molecules are essential in restraining inflammation and resolving infection. They are distinct from immunosuppressive molecules, as they actually promote the body's defense mechanisms against immune and other challenges. SPMs have been shown to inhibit the NLRP3 inflammasome and decrease pro-inflammatory cytokine IL-1b, which can contribute to the cytokine storm seen with some infections.[251]

Aloe vera

Another anti-inflammatory I use often is aloe, mainly because it's one of nature's excellent multitaskers. A succulent plant whose gel has long been used for its sunburn-soothing properties, it can also be used to soothe the epithelium of the gastrointestinal tract in the same manner.[252] The gel, an odorless, clear liquid, is extracted from the innermost part of the leaf and is very safe for long-term use to improve diarrheal symptoms of IBS/IBD and esophagitis. By contrast, the latex of the plant is yellow and bitter and is an irritant/stimulant to the GI tract. This can be useful for sluggish bowels and constipation (see Constipation chapter), although it should be only used for short-term treatment. Because of its additional ability to reduce the reactive oxygen species that can increase inflammation, I utilize this part of the aloe leaf in children who are both inflamed and constipated.

Aloe also has excellent antioxidant properties and has been shown to decrease blood pressure and cholesterol. It improves skin conditions such as acne and psoriasis and continues to be helpful for burns and wounds. For safety and efficacy, aloe should be purchased from a reliable source and certified for its constituents, as each part of the aloe plant is used for drastically different purposes.[253]

Turmeric *Curcuma longa*

Turmeric is another excellent herbal anti-inflammatory. Studies have looked at the use of curcumin to address physical as well as mental health, particularly how it can help with depression and anxiety. This research has concluded that chronic health issues respond well to anti-inflammatories, not only because of the physical improvement these interventions bring but also addressing the depression associated with chronic inflammation as well.[254]

It should be noted that although mainstream media regards turmeric and curcumin as interchangeable, curcumin is, in fact, the main chemical component of the turmeric plant. The Latin name for turmeric is Curcuma longa, which further contributes to the confusion. Although it may seem a matter of semantics, it is important to know that natural supplements created only from dried and ground turmeric root may not provide enough absorption of curcumin and so may not be effective. Curcumin is actually quite a difficult substance to absorb,[255] so it is typically combined with another agent to increase absorption or broken down mechanically in a laboratory to help facilitate its uptake in the body. This is why, historically, turmeric tea is combined with milk, an emulsifier, in "golden milk"—it aids absorption of turmeric's healing constituents. Most commercial products nowadays either utilize phytosome technology[256] (binding the curcumin to phospholipids), wet-milling to create curcumin nanoparticles,[257] or the addition of bioperine[258] (black pepper extract) to enhance absorption. Look for these specialized products for the most effective forms of the herb.

Flavonoids

Next, consider flavonoids, especially quercetin, luteolin, and rutin. These three, in particular, are potent mast cell stabilizers, preventing inflammation or allergies caused by histamine release.[259] Perhaps the most useful of these flavonoids is quercetin, as it is also a zinc ionophore and inhibitor of heat shock proteins needed for viral assembly. It is an excellent preventive and even acute adjunct therapy against viruses.[260]

CBD and Hemp

Finally, an anti-inflammatory we're seeing quite a bit of in the media right now: CBD and hemp oil. Cannabinoids have been shown to suppress pro-inflammatory cytokines, which increase inflammation in the body, particularly in nervous system tissue. It also helps to increase the fox p3 regulatory T cells. Regulatory T (Treg) cells play a central role in the regulation of immune responses to infectious agents, antibodies, allergens, and the commensal microbiota in all of us, including children with PANS/PANDAS.[261] I personally like CBD because not only does it have anti-inflammatory properties, but it has also been shown to decrease OCD[262] and anxiety[263] as well.

Neither CBD nor hemp oil has more than 0.3% of THC, the part of the plant responsible for the "high" (and sometimes anxiety or paranoia) typically associated with marijuana use. Structurally, the primary variance between hemp oil and CBD oil is that hemp oil can only be extracted from a hemp plant. That is not the case with CBD oil, which can be extracted from various plants, including hemp plants, marijuana plants, and select other plants. Both can be successful adjuncts serving the dual purpose of decreasing anxiety and inflammation in our children with PANS/PANDAS. As with all of the interventions I discuss, it is important to work with a qualified practitioner or join our membership program at www.drohara.com to identify quality products.

Gabapentin

Gabapentin has complex mechanisms of action that modestly overlap with other antiepileptics. These mechanisms may include calcium channel-dependent cellular tracking, modulation of GABA biosynthesis, and anti-inflammatory and analgesic effects[264], which impact neurotransmission and overall excitatory tone.[265] Although there is anecdotal evidence of its positive effects on anxiety and those with autoimmune and Basal Ganglia Encephalitis,[266] this off-label use should only be employed by an experienced clinician.[267]

Immunomodulation Based on Symptom Severity

With appropriate therapeutic, nutraceutical, and lifestyle management, most of the children in our practice (up to 80%) do not require more invasive and expensive interventions. The outline below simplifies intervention selection depending on the severity of the disease.[268]

MILD Symptom Severity Treatment

- CBT
- NSAIDs/Ibuprofen
- Herbals, nutraceuticals, and nutrition

MODERATE Symptom Severity Treatment

- As above
- Consider oral steroid trial[269]

MODERATE to SEVERE Symptom Severity Treatment

- As above, including steroid trials

- IVIG[270]

SEVERE to EXTREME Symptom Severity Treatment

- As above, including IVIG[271]

- Therapeutic Plasma Exchange (TPE)[272]

- Rituximab or Mycophenolate mofetil[273]

Oral corticosteroid bursts can dramatically benefit recovery, especially if given within three days of a flare or symptom onset. We will often consider Prednisone 1–2 mg/kg/day, maximum 60–120 mg daily, for five days. Sometimes a patient will improve but then relapse as the effect wanes. In this case, a child may benefit from a more prolonged course followed by taper (for example, Prednisone 2 mg/kg for one week and then taper to 1 mg/kg the second week, 0.5 mg/kg the third week, and 0.5 mg/kg every other day for the final week).[274] Keep in mind that there is a risk that behavioral symptoms may worsen during Prednisone administration, which may be an indication of additional dysbiosis, particularly of yeast.[275]

In moderate to severe cases, IVIG should be considered, as some studies have shown successful amelioration of psychological symptoms of sustained benefit for at least eight weeks and up to 46 weeks with this intervention.[276, 277] Other studies, however, demonstrate no definitive conclusions, either because of limitations of the study or participant number.[278, 279]

Plasmapheresis, also known as therapeutic plasma exchange (TPE), should be considered in severe and extreme cases.[280] Only in rare, extreme cases, especially in those with severe restrictive eating disorders, will we consider Rituximab.[281]

There are a myriad of interventions to consider in the treatment and prevention of children with Basal Ganglia Encephalitis.[282] Great care and understanding are needed in deciding which option is appropriate and warranted for each child. We review and discuss each of these options in our mentoring program. With any child with either abrupt or subacute onset, we should consider using immunomodulatory interventions.[283]

The Addition of Antioxidants

I liken antioxidants to the final piece of the treatment puzzle, as they play a key role in protecting cells from damage from free radicals. Even with the best protocols, inflammation can still wreak havoc on the body, as illness takes time to resolve. Because the brain has a high lipid content, high energy requirements, and weak antioxidant capacity, its cells are especially susceptible to damage by free radicals.[284] Therefore, it is simply not enough to attempt to reduce brain inflammation. We must also provide additional neuroprotection. By definition, free radicals damage cellular tissue, and the newly-generated free radicals from this damage can further destroy cells in an accumulating fashion, creating a snowball effect of mounting inflammation. Antioxidants can help stop this chain reactive process and are essential to an effective anti-inflammatory protocol.[285] The antioxidants I use most often include vitamins A, C, and D, zinc, resveratrol, melatonin, and glutathione.

Vitamin A

Vitamin A enhances the immune system by supporting essential antioxidant functions.[286] We know that deficiency of this vitamin hinders normal regeneration of mucosal barriers previously damaged by infection, in addition to reducing the efficacy of neutrophils, macrophages, and natural killer cells.[287] We also know that this vitamin exhibits mild antiviral action and improves gastrointestinal health by balancing the microbiome,[288] both of which are essential in effectively managing PANS/PANDAS and Basal Ganglia Encephalitis. Some of our children with virally-mediated PANS have evidence of deficiency.[289] In some cases of viral-induced autoimmune encephalitis, I recommend high doses of this vitamin if levels are low. It is important to follow levels, work with a qualified practitioner and understand these encephalitis protocols.[290]

Vitamin C

Like vitamin A, vitamin C is an antioxidant that can be supportive for both prevention of and recovery from infectious disease. This vitamin is remarkable in supporting the epithelial barrier against pathogens, acting as a cofactor for a multitude of antioxidant cascades, and directly affecting the killing of microbes by enhancing the chemotaxis, phagocytosis, and generation of reactive oxygen species in neutrophils and other phagocytic cells.[291, 292] For these reasons, suboptimal levels of vitamin C may result in increased susceptibility to infection.[293] I like to dose vitamin C to the bowel (can exacerbate diarrhea) and behavioral tolerance (can increase agitation), and during illness, starting low and increasing as tolerated to "just below" loose stools. Keep in mind that, unlike vitamins A and D, vitamin C is a water-soluble vitamin and will be excreted rather than becoming toxic, so following levels is not vital.

Vitamin D

The literature demonstrates that vitamin D insufficiency and deficiency are correlated with increased severity of infections.[294, 295, 296] This correlation is seen not only in respiratory infections and overall immune function but also in IBD and other autoimmune disorders.[297] One study also demonstrated that patients with PANDAS have lower levels of 25(OH)D levels than controls and that this deficiency appears to be related to the number of Streptococcal infections and the probability of recurrence.[298]

Vitamin D, as we know, has many different properties with long-reaching effects, including immune modulation,[299] protection of the nervous system,[300] up-regulating gamma-glutamyl transpeptidase,[301] and increasing glutathione.[302] Restoring optimal levels of this antioxidant speeds recovery time from a child's infection, restores immune competence to reduce the severity of future infections, and improves mood. It is cost-effective, fast-acting, and very well tolerated. Patients should utilize the D3 form and take it with K2 as well as fat-containing food for improved bioavailability. As this is a fat-soluble vitamin, levels should be followed.

Zinc

Zinc is important in greater than 300 enzymatic functions, and it inhibits the replication of RNA Type viruses.[303] A 2016 study confirmed that suboptimal levels of zinc are directly correlated with impaired formation, activation, and maturation of lymphocytes, poor cytokine function leading to disrupted intracellular communication, and reduced immunity from improper phagocytosis and oxidative burst.[304] While the recommended dietary allowance (RDA) of zinc for adults is between 8-11 mg daily, it is not uncommon to utilize short-term bursts of the mineral in higher doses during acute infection.[305] When managing chronic infections, such as pneumonia,[306] Lyme disease, and PANS/PANDAS, long-term use of zinc is encouraged and safe, but be aware of its ability to affect copper levels and treat accordingly.[307] Zinc, along with other minerals, may also be vital in improving attention, processing, and overall cognitive function.[308, 309, 310] Monitor zinc through RBC level tests (most accurate measure) and look for signs and symptoms of zinc deficiency, including acne, sparse hair, decreased taste, and white spots or lines on nails (see photo).

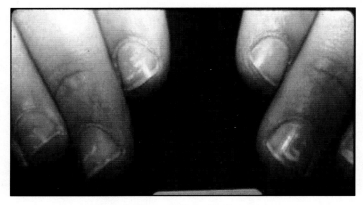

Nails Indicating Zinc Deficiency

Resveratrol

Resveratrol is a potent antioxidant and has been studied as a novel antiviral against coronaviruses.[311] We now know that resveratrol alters the regulation of the renin-angiotensin system and expression of angiotensin-converting enzyme 2, stimulates the immune system, and downregulates pro-inflammatory cytokine release. It also exerts significant antioxidant effects by trapping reactive oxygen species.[312] Although we commonly associate this antioxidant powerhouse with red wine grapes, it is actually most concentrated in *Reynoutria japonica*, or Japanese knotweed. Interestingly, there is increasing evidence of resveratrol's antimicrobial, antifungal, and anti-inflammatory benefits,[313] making it especially well-suited for any infectious disease treatment, especially PANS/PANDAS. Japanese knotweed can help to manage Lyme, Lyme co-infections like Bartonella, and yeast overgrowth; I use it often for all of these.

Melatonin

Melatonin is a hormone that is secreted by our pineal gland, controlling the sleep-wake cycle and is an excellent antioxidant.[314] A study published in 2016[315] succinctly explains its direct detoxification of reactive oxygen and reactive nitrogen species, its ability to stimulate antioxidant enzymes and suppress pro-oxidant enzymes, and its action in Fenton/Haber-Weiss reactions to reduce oxidative stress, and its capacity to resist cellular apoptosis. Utilizing this supplement in children with difficult sleep is fantastic for addressing that specific symptom, but it can also be used solely for its antioxidant properties as well. Lower doses have a sedative effect; higher doses may be needed to optimize antioxidant function against viruses, including COVID-19.[316]

Glutathione

Last but certainly not least is the body's master antioxidant, glutathione.[317] The human body naturally produces glutathione in the liver, but many factors can impact the circulating levels of the antioxidant at any given time. The brain is especially impacted by lower levels of glutathione, as brain cells consume extremely large amounts of oxygen compared to other body cell types. This research has been key in the treatment of understanding the physiologic underpinnings in autism.[318, 319] This means that reactive oxygen species, which are continuously generated during oxygen metabolism, are in high concentrations in the brain. Glutathione is key in the deactivation and removal of these oxidative compounds, supporting mitochondrial function and combating oxidative and physiologic stress in general.[320] When it comes to caring for children with PANS/PANDAS and Basal Ganglia Encephalitis, optimal glutathione levels are needed for the resolution of neuroinflammation and the restoration of brain function. A 2021 study[321] offers new insights into the neuroinflammation and oxidative stress in PANS and the potential role of glutathione in this and other disorders. Of particular note is that some analgesics, including Acetaminophen, deplete glutathione.[322] Thus, using such analgesics at the time of stress, such as post-vaccination, during an active infection, or during bouts of pain, may be counterproductive and, in my opinion, should be curtailed as much as possible. Instead, utilize Ibuprofen or other analgesics. Finally, glutathione may not be as readily absorbed in oral form, so I recommend glutathione gel absorbed buccally or transdermally, nebulized glutathione, intravenous glutathione, or oral NAC which will convert to glutathione in the body.[323] Note that this is a sulfur-containing compound, which may have a noxious smell and taste, so you may have to be creative in your recommendations.

Antioxidants in Food

Antioxidants are a key factor in optimal health and recovery from illness.[324] Although we have discussed individual antioxidants, the best way to prevent disease and treat long-term chronic illness is through an optimal diet and nutrition program.[325] Key antioxidant foods include vegetables such as spinach and broccoli, fruits such as avocados and blueberries, spices such as ginger, garlic, turmeric, and nuts, green tea, and cocoa. For further information, read the next chapter on nutrition and refer to our mentoring program at www.drohara.com.

Nutrition

As any functional medicine practitioner will tell you, treatment of any disease begins in the gut. A substantial amount of what happens in the brain truly begins in the gastrointestinal tract—neurotransmitter production, vitamin, nutrient, and cofactor absorption—so a healthy and balanced microbiome sustained by appropriate diet and nutrition is always the goal.[326] Admittedly, this is easy to say and much harder to implement, especially in children!

Several dietary interventions we discuss for PANS/PANDAS are similar to those for any chronic inflammatory illness.[327] This can make things much easier for parents and caregivers, as an appropriate nutrition plan may not need much individualization once a healthy protocol has been established. Still, individual sensitivities, eating disorders, and food preferences can make mealtimes more challenging, so often, a registered dietician or nutritionist specializing in pediatric neurobehavioral or neurodevelopmental health is a valued care team member. I have been privileged to work with a remarkable dietitian, Vicki Kobliner, MS, RDN, who edited and crafted many of the interventions discussed in this chapter. For more detailed information, I urge you to reach out to our office or an experienced dietitian or nutritionist in your area.

Although there is limited placebo-controlled research regarding specific nutrients and PANS, information and support can certainly be extrapolated from similar conditions, focusing on modulating inflammation, addressing dysbiosis and microbiome health, and targeting specific food restrictions and dietary limitations.[328]

Keep in mind that both the infection associated with PANS or PANDAS, as well as the antibiotics used to treat them, can wreak havoc on a child's gut.[329] The stress of the disease and its treatment (or sometimes lack thereof) negatively impacts the microbiome as well. It follows that both dysbiosis and stress impair immune function, further compromising our "second brains," our GI tracts, and neurological health.[330] Simply put, when you work on improving digestion and the balance of gut flora, you will inevitably have a positive functional effect on immune and nervous system health.

Diet in the Treatment Triad

As we have discussed in other chapters, the treatment of PANS/PANDAS includes three complementary interventions:

1. Removing the source of inflammation (eradicating the pathogen) with antimicrobials

2. Restoring immune competence by decreasing inflammation

3. Treating the symptoms with supportive therapies

Diet can tremendously impact all three of these aspects of care. As with the treatment of all chronic autoimmune diseases, dietary interventions should include:

- Herbs and spices that decrease inflammation and exert antimicrobial properties.

- Nutrient-dense foods that sustain the microbiota and energy needs of the child

- An abundance of unprocessed plant foods, with clean sources of protein and fat to fuel the synthesis of neurotransmitters

- Foods free of inflammatory components and rich in anti-inflammatory compounds.

- For those with reduced appetite/anorexia: higher fat, frequent small meals are ideal.

Herbs and Spices in Our Diets

Anti-Inflammatory

- *Curcuma Longa:* in addition to its anti-inflammatory effects, curcumin has been shown to actively decrease OCD[331] and anxiety.[332]

- *Zingiber Officinalis:* ginger suppresses prostaglandin synthesis through inhibition of cyclooxygenase-1 and cyclooxygenase-2.[333]

- *Allium Sativa:* garlic enhances the immune system by stimulating macrophages, lymphocytes, natural killer (NK) cells, dendritic cells, and eosinophils and modulates cytokine secretion, immunoglobulin production, phagocytosis, and macrophage activation.[334]

- *Cinnamomum spp:* cinnamon reduces LPS-dependent IL-8 secretion in THP-1 monocytes and mitigates the phosphorylation of Akt and $I\kappa B\alpha$.[335]

- *Petroselinum Crispum:* parsley contains phenolic compounds (ferulic acid, gallic acid, and quercetin), which show no evidence of hepatotoxicity or nephrotoxicity and demonstrate remarkable anti-inflammatory activity.[336]

Antimicrobial

- *Origanum Vulgare*: oregano's main constituents, carvacrol, and thymol are responsible for the herb's characteristic odor and antimicrobial and antioxidant activity. These substances work as antibacterial agents to make the cell membrane of pathogens permeable, and the effect is stronger against gram-positive bacteria. In addition, oregano has antioxidant properties effective in retarding the process of lipid peroxidation in fatty foods and scavenging free radicals.[337]

- *Thymus Vulgaris*: like oregano, thyme is high in carvacrol, which is responsible for its antimicrobial and antioxidant activity. Thyme is synergistic with oregano, so the two can be used together for an even greater impact.[338]

- *Cinnamomum spp.:* cinnamon has been shown to inhibit bacteria by damaging their cell membranes, altering the lipid profile, and inhibiting ATPases, cell division, membrane porins, motility, and biofilm formation.[339]

- *Allium Sativa:* In a 2017 study, garlic showed the greatest antimicrobial effect against *Streptococcus mutans* when compared with other preparations individually. The combination of garlic and lemon showed the greatest zone of inhibition in combination with other preparations.[340]

- *Rosmarinus Officinalis:* rosemary extract effectively contributed to in vitro control of important species of microorganisms such as *Candida albicans, Staphylococcus aureus, Enterococcus faecalis, Streptococcus mutans*, and *Pseudomonas aeruginosa* in mono and polymicrobial biofilms.[341]

Nutrient-Rich Foods

In addition to herbs and spices, we must also look at foods high in nutrients needed to decrease anxiety and OCD. These nutrients include zinc, magnesium, iron,[342] omega 3s,[343] and antioxidants such as glutathione,[344] its precursor n-acetyl cysteine, B vitamins,[345] and vitamins C[346] and D.[347]

A Three-Phase Plan for Dietary Changes

Phase One: Clean Up Your Act!

As able, tolerated, and under the direction of a qualified practitioner/dietitian/nutritionist...

1. Remove toxins, including each of the following:

   a. Non-organic products as much as possible

   b. Excess sugar and all sugar substitutes/sweeteners

   c. Synthetic additives, colorings, and preservatives

   d. Animal products that are fed hormones and/or antibiotics

   e. Pesticides

2. Replace and replenish

   a. Bone broth (organic and homemade is best)

   b. "Good" oils (olive, coconut, avocado, macadamia nut)

   c. Fermented foods (cabbage, sauerkraut, non-dairy kefirs, and kombucha)

   d. Anti-inflammatory plants and antimicrobial foods, herbs, and spices (see above)

Phase Two: Reduce Inflammation

Even if a child does not have a known allergy to the following foods, temporary elimination followed by a more long-term reduction of these foods may be beneficial to an anti-inflammatory protocol. Although removal may be the goal, in older children, especially those with eating disorders, any topic of elimination should be done with prudence, full understanding, and compliance with the family, the child, and a registered dietitian or nutritionist.

1. Consider removing gluten

    a. Sensitivities to gluten and actual allergies have been shown to impair cognition, focus, and relatedness and increase inflammation.[348, 349]

    b. The opioid activity of gluten and casein peptides mimic morphine and can act almost like an opiate, inhibiting cysteine uptake and further impacting cognition.[350, 351]

    c. Gluten-containing, processed foods are often high in FODMAPs, oxalates, and lectins, which can also be detrimental.[352]

    d. Gluten interferes[353] with glutamate decarboxylase needed for conversion to GABA, the brain's "zen" neurotransmitter.[354]

2. Consider removing casein (milk protein and all dairy products)

    a. Casein elicits sensitivities and opioid activity similar to gluten[355]

    b. Milk protein sensitivities may also be correlated with autoimmunity[356]

Phase Three: Consider Individualized Diets as Listed Below

1. Remove specific food allergens and sensitivities as able, tolerated, and under the direction of a qualified practitioner/dietitian/nutritionist (keeping in mind that children crave that to which they are most sensitive!).

   a. Accurate food sensitivity testing is challenging at best, so food elimination trials are often the best indicator of food sensitivities and allergies.[357]

   b. Common food sensitivities include soy, peanut, tree nut, egg, fish, shellfish, corn, and banana, but may be found with any foods.

2. Low histamine[358] – histamine levels increase as foods age, so minimizing the following in those with high histamine levels may include:

   a. Aged foods (freeze leftovers instead of refrigerating them)

   b. Fermented foods, cultured foods

   c. Tomatoes, eggplant, spinach (all nightshade vegetables)

3. Low Glutamate – Excitotoxins may cause excess neurotransmission in the brain and can lead to brain inflammation.[359]

   a. Food sources include MSG, hydrolyzed proteins, natural flavors, peas, mushrooms, tomatoes, bone broth, and cheeses.

   b. Consider countering exposure to these glutamate-rich foods with "anti-glutamates," including pycnogenol, rosemary, lemon balm, chamomile, and foods high in magnesium, taurine, GABA, and L-theanine.[360]

4. Low Phenols/Salicylates[361] – FAILSAFE diet eliminates the following:

    a. Artificial food additives, colorings, preservatives.

    b. Salicylates and polyphenolic foods and medications, including many fruits and vegetables.

    c. Aromatic chemicals are found in perfumes, cleaning products, personal care, and candles.

    d. Medications such as COX-II inhibitors.

5. Low Oxalates are molecules that link with minerals (particularly calcium) and crystallize, increasing or exacerbating inflammation.[362] Oxalate absorption increases greatly with compromised GI function (or "leaky gut").

    a. Foods high in oxalates may need to be minimized, including nuts such as almonds and leafy greens such as spinach.

    b. Low concentrations of *Lactobacillus* in the microbiota reduce oxalate degradation, causing high oxalate absorption, so supplementation with these probiotics is helpful.[363]

    c. Low vitamin B6 and sulfur also result in excess oxalates.[364]

    d. Calcium citrate can bind to oxalates to excrete them from the gut.

6. SCD/GAPS – Specific Carbohydrate Diet[365]/Gut and Psychology Syndrome Diet.[366]

    a. Removal of all grains and complex sugars that can ferment in the gut and feed yeast and other germs.

    b. Both of these diets emphasize protein, veggies, fruits, and healthy fats, with a controlled amount of nuts and nut flours.

c. Diets exclude all di- and polysaccharides.

7. Mediterranean Diet,[367] Modified Paleo, or Autoimmune Paleo anti-inflammatory protocols designed to heal intestinal inflammation and reduce symptoms of autoimmunity

   a. Eliminate all processed foods, grains, xylitol, stevia, mannitol, dried fruit, eggs, gums, nightshades, tapioca, alcohol, chocolate, and dairy products.

   b. Support the healthy use of proteins, oils, fresh vegetables, and fruits.

Dietitians/Nutritionists as Part of the Care Team

Balancing a child's food restrictions and preferences with nutritional adequacy while keeping parents' sanity at the top of their minds is challenging, and I find that it is often necessary to include the expertise of a knowledgeable dietitian or nutritionist on the child's care team. Look for those who have experience with eating disorders and food sensitivities in children, and reach out to our clinic for possible local referrals. It is essential to build a team. It takes a variety of interventions and a village to care for our children and families. Nutrition is a key factor in this care if done with expertise and accommodation to each child's and family's needs.

As mentioned, it is essential to understand, appropriately assess, and then manage eating disorders, keeping in mind that an abrupt onset of food restrictions can be a manifestation of PANS/PANDAS in 20% of cases.[368] Also, as you may have experienced, creating an effective nutrition plan for children with PANS/PANDAS or other autoimmune diseases beyond a general "anti-inflammatory diet" can be overwhelming, and it is compounded with the risk of limiting foods, as this can bring about or exacerbate symptoms of anorexia and OCD.[369]

Particularly in children with eating disorders, families should work with their therapists to avoid and treat additional food-related OCD issues, in addition to a registered dietitian or nutritionist.[370]

STEP 3: SYMPTOM - SPECIFIC TREATMENT

Anxiety

Tics

Obsessive-Compulsive Disorder (OCD)

Brain Fog

Sleep

Constipation

Neurotherapy

Note: further guidance on treatment, including dosages and preferred brands, is available through membership and mentorship options at www.drohara.com.

ANXIETY

Anxiety is a common and debilitating symptom for children with PANS/PANDAS and Basal Ganglia Encephalitis. It often underlies the most common presenting symptoms of OCD, tics, and brain fog. The anxiety accompanying PANS/PANDAS can take on many forms, including a seven-year-old child washing his hands continuously out of fear of germs, a sixteen-year-old suddenly terrified of the dark or of having nightmares and now needing to sleep with a parent, or a twelve-year-old suddenly preoccupied with choking and therefore severely restricting food intake. The types of anxiety that can present are endless and are usually motivated by a single or multiple irrational and misunderstood or subconscious fears.

Treating Anxiety in PANS/PANDAS

Because anxiety is at the heart of PANS/PANDAS and has overlapped with many of the other classic symptoms of the disease, many of the interventions discussed in other chapters, especially on OCD and tics, are also mentioned here. Still, a few nuances should be noted when considering anxiety as a standalone symptom, as noted below.

Pharmaceutical Management

Most physicians choose to use Selective Serotonin Reuptake Inhibitors (SSRIs) to lessen the intensity of anxiety symptoms, and although these can be helpful, there can also be side effects.[371] For this reason, I prefer starting with herbal medicine and nutraceuticals to manage anxiety, as there can be multiple benefits with minimal to no side effects. Still, if a patient seems a good candidate for prescription SSRIs or Serotonin and Norepinephrine Reuptake Inhibitors (SNRIs), consider the following guidelines as a starting point.

Start at a very low dosage and slowly titrate up, as many children will do well with lower doses.[372] Especially in children with Autism Spectrum Disorder, some research shows that the side effects of utilizing high doses of SSRIs, particularly with children experiencing inflammation in the brain, may outweigh the benefits with reports of behavioral activation—specifically, increased activity, impulsivity, and insomnia. I have also seen this kind of activation in children with PANS/PANDAS and share this with my families so that they can decide whether or not to proceed with increased dosing of SSRIs.[373]

Some of our children also have situational anxiety, performance anxiety, or social anxiety. Many of these children will improve with Propranolol, a beta-blocker that has been shown to help with generalized anxiety and its peripheral symptoms, including tachycardia and sweating. I often will trial this prescriptive medication at the beginning of treatment because it is usually well-tolerated and has few side effects.[374] Propranolol is also helpful in treating dysautonomia or POTS (Postural Orthostatic Tachycardia Syndrome) seen often in children with chronic illness, including more chronic or severe cases of autoimmune encephalitis (AE).[375]

Natural Interventions

Adaptogenic and Nervine Herbs

At the top of my list of first-line interventions are nervine and adaptogenic herbs, which are plant-based medicines used to support the nervous system and tonify the adrenal glands, respectively. Adaptogens can help our children appropriately react to or recover from both short-term and long-term physical or mental stress and can help to alleviate fatigue, enhance mental performance, and ease depression and anxiety.[376] Nervines and adaptogens that I use frequently include *Withania somnifera* (ashwagandha, also known as the "herbal valium"),[377] *Rhodiola rosea*,[378] *Melissa officinalis* (lemon balm),[379] *Passiflora incarnata* (passion flower),[380] *Ocimum tenuiflorum* (holy basil),[381] *Glycyrrhiza glabra* (licorice root),[382] and the mushroom *Cordyceps militaris*.[383]

B Vitamins

B vitamins can also be useful in decreasing anxiety. The most important of these are derivatives of folate, including folinic acid and MTHF or "methylated folate." In children with diagnosed MTHFR C677 defects[384] or Cerebral Folate Deficiency (CFD),[385] higher doses of folinic acid or 5-MTHF metabolites may be required for the child to actually utilize this vitamin effectively.

Other B vitamins, such as pyridoxine (B6), niacin (B5), and even a general "B complex," may nourish the adrenal glands, which in turn supports a normal and healthy stress response.[386] Some practitioners utilize B6 in combination with magnesium to balance anxiety, though I prefer to use magnesium alone. Lastly, although often referred to as a B vitamin, inositol (erroneously nicknamed "vitamin B8") is an important calmative nutrient to consider. It heightens the activity of serotonin and can have a vital role in mood, anxiety, OCD, and emotional balance in appropriate dosages.[387]

Minerals

As previously noted, minerals such as magnesium also reduce anxiety. A 2017 review that looked at 18 different studies found that magnesium reduced anxiety and improved brain function by regulating neurotransmitters.[388] For those who do not experience constipation, I recommend magnesium glycinate or malate and will sometimes use magnesium threonate if sleep or brain fog is also an issue. I use magnesium oxide and citrate as needed and tolerated for those children with constipation, as it reduces bowel transit time.[389] Too much magnesium can result in diarrhea or loose stools, so following RBC magnesium may be helpful and necessary in maintaining safe magnesium levels.

Amino Acids

Another natural substance I have found much success with is gamma-aminobutyric acid (GABA). Research studies in both animals and humans show that GABA has an important role in the amygdala, modulating anxiety-related behaviors.[390] This complements research investigating other neurotransmitters in the amygdala that have been implicated in modulating anxiety, including serotonin, opioid peptides, endocannabinoids,[391] and oxytocin.[392] GABA is an inexpensive, readily available over-the-counter product with low risk.[393] I particularly like using GABA in combination with the calming amino acid theanine, as they promote relaxation and restful sleep.[394] Adding theanine boosts brain levels of GABA and other calming brain chemicals, including serotonin and dopamine, safely and effectively.

Lifestyle Changes

Just as with adults, exercise and meditation are essential to reducing anxiety. Through the natural release of endorphins, regular aerobic exercise is associated with the lower sympathetic nervous system and hypothalamic-pituitary-adrenal (HPA) axis reactivity.[395] Meditation, the practice of focused concentration and continually bringing yourself back to the present, also addresses stress and reduces anxiety. As a medical doctor, I have no authority in either of these fields, but I practice them myself. Please review the Neurotherapy chapter for more information.

A Note on Rage

Rage, aggression, and agitation can also be some of the first indications of autoimmune encephalitis of the basal ganglia. Such symptoms, like most of those with this disorder, come on suddenly and dramatically. The rage and aggression can be so severe that parents are afraid and uncertain about how to proceed, sometimes calling in the police or EMS for assistance. Some children do not remember the rage episode. They may exhibit remorse, but they do not really know what they did or even remember the behaviors.

Like many of the other symptoms, we have described in this guidebook, treating these can be very difficult for parents, but should first begin by determining and then treating the underlying cause, such as antibiotics for Mycoplasma or Strep, managing the inflammation, and finally focusing on the individual symptoms. The same interventions described in treating tics, anxiety, and OCD can be applied to treating rage, aggression, and agitation, as they may be interrelated.

Of note, in addition to the previously mentioned infectious triggers of autoimmune encephalitis, children with rage should also be assessed for Bartonella, a Lyme co-infection that ticks and cat scratches or bites can transmit. In addition to rage and anxiety, typical symptoms of Bartonella infection include long bone and muscle pain, foot pain (particularly the soles of the feet), visual disturbances, and purple, blanching stretch marks or streaks that do not follow dermal lines. Please review our section on Lyme for more information on Bartonella and other Lyme Co-infections.

Tics

In addition to anxiety, OCD, brain fog, and rage, tics can be a symptom of sudden onset in our children with PANS/PANDAS and Basal Ganglia Encephalitis. Tics are involuntary and uncontrolled repetitive movements or sounds. Motor tics often involve blinking, throat clearing or sniffing, mouth or facial movements, head twitching, shoulder shrugging, or other simple and sudden body movements. Complex tics can also involve bending to touch the floor, large arm or truncal movements, or more intricate uncontrolled actions. Vocal tics are involuntary expressions that can include noises, grunts, or repetitive words (sometimes obscenities) or phrases.[396] Tics can be temporary or long-lasting, such as Tourette's Syndrome (TS).

It is important to be able to differentiate between the tics of PANS/PANDAS and those of TS, as management may be very different. Tourette's Syndrome is defined as:[397]

- two or more motor tics and at least one vocal tic, although they might not always happen at the same time

- having had tics for at least a year

- having tics that begin before age 18 years

- having symptoms that are not a result of taking drugs, pharmaceutical or otherwise, or of having another medical condition, such as seizures, Huntington's disease, or post viral or other autoimmune encephalitis

While they may seem quite similar to tics associated with Tourette's Syndrome, those resulting from PANS/PANDAS are hallmarked by *abrupt onset*. They seem to come on dramatically, and most caregivers will describe the change as "almost overnight."

This distinction is very important. Although some aspects of the conventional treatment for Tourette's Syndrome overlap, such as Cognitive Behavioral Therapy and relaxation techniques, some of the more common pharmaceuticals prescribed for the condition would, at best, mask the underlying pathology and, at worse, exacerbate the already complicated health picture. A functional approach to treating the tics associated with PANS/PANDAS is often "covered" by the treatments targeting other PANS/PANDAS symptoms, so it does not always need a separate intervention. Finding the root cause and addressing foundational health first is essential. Investigating and treating Strep, Mycoplasma, viruses, yeast/mold, Lyme, and co-infections (especially Bartonella), as well as metabolic triggers such as anesthesia and pesticide exposure, are essential to successfully treating the abrupt onset of any of these symptoms.

Treating Tics

Natural Medicine

Magnesium

In the realm of vitamins and minerals, magnesium is a powerful natural intervention to help allay tics. Some children with tics triggered by autoimmune encephalitis have less than optimal magnesium levels. While not quite at "deficiency" status, magnesium insufficiency is very real and can be very serious, leading to musculoskeletal pain, constipation, and a heightened sense of anxiety.[398]

Start with the diet first, if possible. Some of my favorite magnesium-rich foods include almonds, Brazil nuts, pumpkin and sunflower seeds, spinach, avocados, and even dark chocolate. Chocolate almond butter smoothies with a handful of spinach thrown in for good measure work wonders for less adventurous eaters! Our chapter on diet and nutrition and our mentoring program on nutrition and autoimmune encephalitis can provide other fun and effective dietary concepts and recipes.

Often children with tics require more magnesium than can be found with nutritional interventions alone. Magnesium glycinate is quite gentle on the gastrointestinal tract and fairly well absorbed, so that it may be a good initial supplement choice. If a child is constipated, consider magnesium citrate, a sometimes more irritating but cleansing preparation, to improve both bowel function and increase magnesium stores. If brain fog and memory seem to be an issue, magnesium threonate might be a good choice, as this form has been shown to calm the brain more specifically. Magnesium taurate and magnesium oxide can also be good choices, depending on the child's presentation, including Autism.[399] Dosing depends on the weight and age of the child, as well as blood levels (RBC magnesium and ionized calcium), which should be periodically checked.

Finally, other administration forms, such as IV and topical, can also be considered.[400] Because magnesium is well absorbed through the skin, Epsom salt (magnesium sulfate) baths are often included in my treatment plans for children averse to taking oral medicines. Magnesium baths combined with baking soda can promote healthy detoxification. Adding one-half to one cup of each to a warm bath just before bed can become a soothing part of a family's nighttime routine. The calming bath helps to induce a good night's sleep, which is critical for not only everyone's sanity but also for restorative detoxification support. If a child does not take baths, this can also be done in a foot bath or in a spray bottle (putting one-quarter to one-half cup of Epsom salt in a large spray bottle of water) and using this during a shower or after a swim or exercise.

CBD

Cannabidiols, especially hemp oil, can help decrease tics and manage inflammation and anxiety, as described in other chapters. Although it is expected that cannabis may help any anxiety-based disease, cannabis has been shown to specifically reduce motor and verbal tics due to Tourette's (and, by extension, PANS/PANDAS).[401] As this intervention has gained in popularity, there are hundreds of brands available to consumers, each featuring varying amounts of CBD, THC, or full-spectrum cannabinoids. It is essential to work with a qualified practitioner and utilize a trusted, researched, and effective brand to safely administer this supplement.

Nutraceuticals and Herbs

N-acetyl cysteine, or NAC, as discussed in greater detail in our chapter on OCD, is a "semi-essential" amino acid, meaning the body makes some amount naturally. Still, it must also be consumed in the diet to maintain optimal levels. This amino acid increases glutathione, promotes natural detoxification and antioxidant support and is also an important respiratory tract decongestant. As with OCD, research shows that NAC, at doses of 600-2700 mg daily (depending on age, weight, and symptoms), can alleviate anxiety[402] and tics.[403]

Other remedies to consider with tics include the following:

- GABA (gamma-aminobutyric acid): is an inhibitory neurotransmitter that helps to reduce neuronal excitation and excitability.[404] Because exogenous GABA does not easily cross the blood-brain barrier, L-theanine can often help its transport.[405]

- Adaptogens, such as ashwagandha and rhodiola, help to alleviate adrenal stress, which may impact the occurrence of tics (refer to chapter on Anxiety for more information and research)

- Methylated folate, especially in those with Cerebral Folate Deficiency or significant MTHFR defects (refer to chapter on Anxiety for more information and research)

- Calming agents and sleep aides such as valerian,[406] chamomile,[407] and passion flower (also refer to chapter on Anxiety for more information and research)

Pharmaceuticals

In addition to the foundational interventions that reduce inflammation and stabilize brain function discussed in other chapters, consider these targeted medicines. Antihypertensives can help in multiple forms: alpha-blockers like Clonidine[408] and Guanfacine[409] can help reduce tics and help with ADHD symptoms, and beta-blockers such as Inderal and Propranolol can reduce tics and anxiety, as well as confounding symptoms of dysautonomia (more in the Anxiety chapter).

Neuroleptics or antipsychotics such as Risperidone, Pimozide, or Aripiprazole can be used, too. A 2011 study found Risperidone as effective as Haloperidol in treating tics. It may also effectively treat PANS/PANDAS comorbidities like obsessive-compulsive and aggressive symptoms.[410] Keep in mind that side effects for this entire class of drugs include drowsiness, shakiness, weight gain, blurred vision, dry mouth, constipation, and exacerbation of twitches, as in tardive dyskinesia. Discuss these negative effects with families before prescribing to manage expectations better. As always, start low and increase slowly, only as tolerated and necessary.[411]

Anticonvulsants such as Levetiracetam are usually used to treat partial-onset, tonic-clonic, and myoclonic seizures but can also be used to decrease tics. It may be necessary to order an EEG in children with tics before considering an anticonvulsant for treatment.[412]

SSRIs such as Sertraline and Fluoxetine have been used in the past but often do not specifically address tics. If they are not helpful in other ways, such as reducing anxiety, they may only cause sedation and can even exacerbate tics. For these reasons, this class of drugs is not among my top picks to consider for tics associated with PANS/PANDAS.[413]

Movement disorder treatments like Tetrabenazine affect dopamine, serotonin, and norepinephrine levels in the brain. Although this drug is most often used in people with Huntington's Disease or other conditions with rapid repetitive movements, it has also been shown to improve motor and vocal tics.[414]

Lastly, Botox. Experimentation on Botulinum toxin injections' effects on movement disorders predates its use in cosmetic medicine, and multiple decades of research have shown these injections into the eyelids, neck, and vocal cords can reduce uncontrollable winking, blinking, head shaking, and vocalizations. Although these are not licensed uses for branded Botulinum toxin injections, they may be administered by an experienced practitioner with a signed informed consent. The effect is transient, lasting up to 3 months, but may still be worth consideration in select patients.[415]

Lifestyle Factors and Complementary Therapies

Diet

"Food is medicine" is a theme of our practice and goes well beyond treating tics, OCD, anxiety, or any of the behaviors or symptoms we discuss in this guidebook. Healthy eating is important for the entire family. Eating as many whole, unprocessed, unrefined foods as possible is critical. A diet high in healthy oils, vegetables, fruits, and protein is key, but a diet high in protein can be especially important for children with tics. Encourage meals that include meats, eggs, nuts, seeds, and even protein powders if necessary. Children in my practice have found significant benefits with chicken, beef, and calves' liver, and our families have found creative ways to get them to eat it! Our mentoring program includes recipes and handouts with multiple kinds of wonderful suggestions.

One key nutrient in a protein-rich diet is choline. This essential nutrient can decrease tics by supporting the growth and myelination of brain cells, producing phospholipids (a major component of cell membranes), and making acetylcholine (to support mood, memory, and muscle control), and encouraging methylation as a precursor to betaine. The best source of choline is eggs, but if your child is intolerant of eggs, consider other animal protein sources, such as brussels sprouts, cauliflower, and nut butter, to meet choline needs.[416]

In general, we want to focus on foods that actively decrease inflammation and minimize foods that can exacerbate it, such as gluten, dairy, eggs, corn, high fructose corn syrups, and artificial chemicals, colorings, and additives. Often elimination diets are the best way to figure out if a food may be exacerbating a child's symptoms. Although testing can be done to identify and address food allergies, intolerances, and sensitivities, elimination trials are a cost-effective, more accurate, and truly effective way to pinpoint foods that may be exacerbating a child's tics. Elimination diets involve removing one food or category of food for a period of time to see how symptoms are impacted and reintroducing it carefully, often in an overindulgence or "pig-out," to confirm its impact on sensitivities. Of course, with true IgE allergies, RAST or skin testing may be necessary, and a pig-out is not appropriate or safe. Thus, it is important to ensure that you and your families understand the difference between IgE allergies and IgG sensitivities or intolerances when discussing and attempting elimination diets and reintroduction. The elimination period for food sensitivities and intolerances is often one to two weeks, but for dairy, it should be three weeks, and for gluten, three months.[417]

Tips for a successful elimination diet:

- Keep a meticulous food diary/log to track effects and responses.

- Be aware that as tics may wax and wane, it may take a few attempts of removing and reintroducing food to determine its effect on symptoms.

- After the period of elimination, especially if you are not sure if the removal helped, overindulge on the offending food (we're talking two to three servings per day for two to three days) when you reintroduce it to see if this aggravates the tics. This is the pig-out phase!

- If you find no change in symptoms when you remove the food and no aggravation when you reintroduce it, then this food or category is most likely not a factor for that child.

- With any concerns about eating disorders, be extremely cautious with elimination trials or diets and work with a qualified practitioner.

Therapy

I would highly recommend working with a therapist trained in dealing with children with tics, particularly a Cognitive Behavioral Therapist (CBT). Please refer to the Neurotherapy chapter and our mentorship program for more information. As a practitioner and parent myself, I can recommend some helpful therapeutic tips I have picked up along the way, such as:

- As much as possible, reduce stress, anxiety, boredom, and most especially, fatigue. A good night's sleep is critical!

- Ignore tics as much as possible; focusing on them only accentuates the stress and involuntary movements. Do not punish tics or use bribery to try to control them.

- On the other hand, do not "feed the beast." A child does not get a pass on chores or household or school responsibilities because of their tics, anxiety, or OCD.

- Reassure the family and the child. Do not blame or shame a child with tics.

- Let teachers, coaches, and other adults know about tics so they're aware of them and know how to react or not to react when they occur.

Countering Tics

Replace or counter tics with appropriate interventions, such as playing the drums (you'll be pleased to learn that there are electric and soft drum pads to minimize the noise), chewing gum, humming, or whistling. Engaging in intentional activities that keep your hands busy, such as knitting and hand play (as with squeezing stress balls or finger knitting), can help engage children and minimize tics.

Electromagnetic Frequency

Consider reducing EMF exposure and decreasing computer and electronic use as much as possible. Even minimal use of electronics or exposure to WiFi can aggravate a sensitive child, and tics can be impacted greatly by areas high in electromagnetic radiation. When using electronic devices, we encourage families to reduce exposure to stimulating blue light by wearing blue-light-blocking glasses and to consider utilizing well-researched EMF protective products. For further information, see www.ewg.org.

Acupuncture

Acupuncture is founded on the concept that the body's life force, or *qi*, flows freely in healthy individuals. When there is illness or imbalance, the pathways *qi* follows, known as meridians, are blocked. Unblocking them by stimulating meridian access points through acupuncture or acupressure is an excellent way to naturally rebalance a child's energy.[418] As with any practitioner or intervention discussed, look for a licensed practitioner (LAc) who has experience with children and who can individualize treatment.

Meditation/Mindfulness and Hypnosis

I have found particular success with teaching children breathing techniques, slow and intentional alternating nasal breathing, mantras, and other forms of relaxation and stress management. Hypnosis is another behavioral approach that can help a child to identify the triggers and urges that precede a tic. Hypnosis can teach patients how to control and prevent and gain control over the tics. Learn more in the Neurotherapy chapter.

Physical Medicine

Massage or intentional muscle relaxation with heat can be soothing to overused and tense muscles and can increase serotonin and dopamine while decreasing cortisol, thereby reducing tics. Exercise is essential for overall health, especially outdoor activity. Moderate level exercise has been shown to decrease the severity of the tics.[419] An exercise program that stretches and increases flexibility in overworked muscles can help alleviate some of the pain brought on by tics.[420]

Homeopathy

Lastly, I recommend working with a practitioner familiar with classical homeopathy to determine the correct remedy for a child's unique presentation. Although OTC combination remedies and homeopathic detoxification kits may be helpful, one may only truly see benefits from homeopathy when working with a trained homeopath who can individualize and optimize this form of treatment. Because homeopathy peels back medical complexities layer by layer, exacerbations and healing crises may occur. A knowledgeable homeopath should guide caregivers to determine what is healthy and normal and what needs further attention.

Obsessive-Compulsive Disorder (OCD)

Obsessive-Compulsive Disorder, "OCD," is a complex group of symptoms that includes ritualistic or perseverative behaviors that must be repeated in order to control fears or anxieties.[421] OCD behaviors can include obsessions with any or several of the following:

- Washing: usually because of a fear of contamination from germs or a fear of becoming dirty or sick.

- Hoarding: finding it hard to discard anything or determine items unnecessary.

- Doubting: involving a strong fear of being wrong, rejected, or blamed to the point of an inability to do something for fear of being ridiculed or found incorrect.

- Checking: checking rooms, appliances, and anything repeatedly because of a fear of being harmed by perceived dangers such as fire, accidents, robbery, or animals.

- Counting: tending to perseverate on numbers and the overwhelming need to count or repetitively do something in a certain order or a certain number of times.

- Arranging: fixating on order, patterns, symmetry, or balance.

As previously discussed, many children with OCD may have intrusive thoughts and mental compulsions. These children try very hard to hide these intrusive thoughts. As practitioners, we may not identify physical compulsions or even see these mental compulsions. It is important to listen intently to the child, caregivers, and even your office staff to identify Obsessive-Compulsive Disorders correctly.

OCD can be a challenging behavior for families to navigate because it is not well understood, is not logical, and requires the family to adjust much of their routines and expectations to accommodate. In addition, it may bring up feelings of anxiety, frustration, sadness, or guilt in caregivers and other family members, creating even more barriers to connecting with appropriate help.

Deeper than the Diagnosis

It is simply not enough to diagnose a child with OCD and use pharmaceuticals and therapy to treat it. Although therapy and medication are important aspects of a successful plan, functional medicine requires us to look into the actual cause of the child's OCD. We find that in addition to the abrupt onset of OCD with PANS/PANDAS, the condition can be caused by other infectious or autoimmune triggers, oxidative stress, genetic polymorphisms, glutamatergic abnormalities, or other abnormalities of neurotransmission. Though the list seems extensive, each of these should be carefully considered in examining OCD. However, remember that an *abrupt* onset of OCD or other symptoms is such a distinctive sign of PANS/PANDAS and Basal Ganglia Encephalitis that it is almost always the culprit. In fact, more than 80% of cases of abrupt onset OCD have evidence of postinfectious neuroinflammation in the caudate/putamen and basal ganglia.[422] Still, practitioners must also rule out other forms of encephalitis or cerebral vasculitis, tumors, strokes, physical or sexual abuse, psychological or physical trauma, as well as exposure to toxins, medications, or illicit drugs, before concluding that PANS/PANDAS is the solitary trigger.[423]

Treatment

Treatment of OCD should always include therapy, especially Cognitive Behavioral Therapy (CBT), Dialectical Behavioral Therapy (DBT), or sometimes Exposure and Response Prevention (ERP). Further discussion can be found in our Neurotherapy Chapter and our mentorship program.

Pharmaceuticals

As mentioned previously, pharmaceutical management of OCD can be very helpful and often includes antidepressants, anti-anxiety medications, or other classes of medications, such as SSRIs or SNRIs, including Citalopram, Escitalopram, Fluvoxamine, Fluoxetine, Paroxetine, Sertraline, and Clomipramine as well as Duloxetine and Venlafaxine.[424] I have found that if any of these medications are considered, often very low doses titrated up slowly work best. All side effects should be discussed and monitored, including:

- Nausea or stomach upset
- Inability to sit still
- Sleepiness or insomnia
- A heightened sense of energy
- Drowsiness
- Dry mouth
- Racing heart (requiring EKG monitoring)
- Concentration problems

- Problems with urination

- Weight gain

Although these treatments are standard in OCD care, I have found many natural interventions to be both safe and helpful for children with neurobehavioral issues and OCD. I will often utilize these first.

Natural Treatments

Herbal Medicine

As discussed in the chapter on Anxiety, herbal interventions to consider for OCD include adrenal adaptogens such as *Withania somnifera* (Ashwagandha), often referred to as the "herbal Valium," and *Rhodiola rosea*. As calmative, non-stimulating herbs, these particular adaptogens can help with perseverative behaviors, anxiety, and OCD while promoting neurocognitive balance. Ashwagandha, in particular, has been shown in mice models to decrease OCD behaviors comparably to Fluoxetine.[425] This herb helps the body to more effectively deal with stress, promoting better mood and energy regulation. It can be helpful for children with yeast overgrowth and those with thyroid issues, as it exerts mild antifungal[426] properties and increases thyroid hormone levels by decreasing cortisol.[427]

The nervine herb *Passiflora incarnata* (passionflower) has been shown to reduce perceived stress, impacting many symptoms which develop from increased stress load, including anxiety, OCD, depression, and insomnia.[428] Clinically, we see this improving OCD as well. A 2001 study reported that passionflower managed anxiety and OCD as well as the benzodiazepine drug Oxazepam without the problematic side effects.[429]

CBD and hemp oil can also be an excellent intervention for children with OCD symptoms in PANS/PANDAS. Cannabidiols decrease inflammation and pain signaling, improving anxiety, OCD, and depression. In fact, in a 2021 study, patients reported a 60% reduction in compulsions, a 49% reduction in intrusions, and a 52% reduction in anxiety from before to after inhaling cannabis.[430] They have also been shown to reverse anti-compulsive effects and OCD behaviors such as marble burying in mice.[431] Because of its dual effect of decreasing inflammation and pain as well as decreasing anxiety and OCD, it is often a good early treatment choice.

Nutraceuticals

One of my first choices in the natural treatment of OCD is n-acetyl cysteine (NAC). NAC is a nutritional supplement that enhances glutathione S-transferase activity and stimulates glutathione biosynthesis. It is a potent antioxidant, promoting detoxification and mitochondrial membrane support. Multiple studies have shown the relationship between OCD, oxidative stress, and altered glutathione metabolism. Like sulforaphane, as a glutathione precursor, NAC has been shown to have multiple purposes, including decreasing OCD,[432] tics, and anxiety. Published studies report its treatment of trichotillomania,[433] compulsive gambling,[434] nail-biting,[435] obsessive excoriation, and skin picking.[436] One caveat for NAC: the amino acid is easily oxidized when exposed to air and is often more bioavailable when buffered and individually packaged. Because technology is rapidly changing, do your due diligence in finding updated formulations for best absorption or instruct patients to individually blister pack each daily dose of n-acetyl cysteine.

Although commonly known as "vitamin B8," inositol is not a vitamin but rather a beneficial sugar that influences insulin response and exerts effects on mood and cognition. This intervention has been shown to decrease OCD through its effect on serotonin,[437] although high doses (up to 18 grams) may be required to see an appreciable effect.

5-HTP, lithium orotate, and GABA can also decrease obsessive-compulsive behaviors and calm, repetitive thoughts. 5-HTP, an amino acid and precursor of serotonin, raises levels of this neurotransmitter effectively, which decreases somatic symptoms like insomnia and also calms OCD symptoms. Because of its mechanism of action, 5-HTP should not be taken with SSRIs, as it may cause an excess of serotonin.[438] Lithium orotate may cross the blood-brain barrier more easily than lithium salts typically prescribed, so low doses may be quite effective without unwanted side effects like dulled personality, memory loss, or weight gain that are seen with prescriptive Lithium.[439,440] Finally, Gamma-Aminobutyric Acid (GABA) levels in patients with OCD are significantly lower than in those not living with the condition.[441] Research is now focusing on how GABA supplementation can improve OCD symptoms by restoring normal GABA levels. We find clinically that each of these may help to calm the brain, decreasing excitability, anxiety, and OCD.

Minerals

Vitamin and mineral insufficiency can greatly impact children and adults with OCD. I pay special attention to low levels of selenium, zinc, iron, and magnesium, as well as higher levels of calcium. Optimal levels of magnesium and zinc, in particular, are associated with optimal brain function (and therefore decreased OCD). We know that magnesium deficiency can cause hyperactivity, anxiety, twitching, and tics, not to mention its effects on insomnia and constipation.[442] Zinc deficiency can lead to problems with energy metabolism and immunity, as well as acne, mouth sores, spotted lines on nails, and loss of smell and taste.[443]

Lifestyle Factors

In all children with OCD and anxiety, lifestyle factors should be addressed, focusing on sleep (addressed in another chapter), exercise, and mindfulness training. Mindfulness involves paying attention to the present internally and externally without being *hooked* or *entangled* by thoughts. Mindfulness can include simple mantras (even repeating a favorite song!), breathing awareness, movement (yoga or stretching), grounding (body awareness), and visual, sound, and taste awareness exercises. Refer to the Anxiety, Tics, and Neurotherapy chapters for more information.

Nutrition and GI Health

The health of the gastrointestinal tract is at the core of nearly every neurobehavioral issue I see. The association between constipation and encopresis with repetitive, ritualistic, and compulsive behaviors such as OCD, anxiety, and sensory over-responsivity is incredibly compelling.[444] I firmly believe that treating dysbiosis or germ overgrowth of any sort is paramount to successful outcomes. This is done through the use of antimicrobials (see Step 1: Eradicate the Pathogen) in addition to an anti-inflammatory diet specifically tailored to each child's dietary needs and restrictions.[445]

Brain Fog

Processing issues and problems with mental acuity are common in children with PANS/PANDAS and Basal Ganglia Encephalitis. Many children, families, and teachers refer to this confusion as "brain fog." Often, auditory and visual processing delays, difficulties with attention and focus, and executive function deficits are present.

Brain fog is really a "grab bag" term for any inability to attend, concentrate, or learn and is a hallmark of PANS/PANDAS and Basal Ganglia Encephalitis. It can be associated with or caused by lack of sleep, intrusive or off-topic thoughts, anxiety, or mood swings–even an acute onset of OCD. Although there is no data on the percentage of children with brain fog, as it encompasses so many different aspects of thinking and focusing, we do know that in several studies,[446] up to 90% of children have difficulty concentrating, 80-85% have sleep disturbances that can lead to difficulties attending in school, 70% have abrupt onset of hyperactivity as in ADHD, 70% have inattentiveness as in ADD, and 60% will have various learning difficulties or memory loss. It is clear that "brain fog" can take on many forms. A trained neuropsychologist can help differentiate in an individual child what specific executive function defects, memory issues, attention problems, or other processing difficulties a child may be experiencing. This evaluation can help guide the specific educational accommodations a child may require.

It is important to remember that PANS and PANDAS have an episodic course, so fluidity within the school setting is vital. A child that can be on time to class, attend an entire lecture, and access information one day may be unable to master one or more of the skills the next. Thus, understanding the relapsing and remitting course of this disease is essential for parents and practitioners, educators, and all school personnel.

In addition to the above issues, children who feel "out of it" or who describe themselves as having "brain fog" may also be experiencing one or many of the following abrupt onset symptoms:

- Dysgraphia, clumsiness, or trouble with handwriting.

- Margin drift and left-sided neglect in right-handed children when writing or drawing.

- Sensory modulation issues such as insensitivity or hypersensitivity.

- Tics (which in and of themselves can be very fatiguing to the body and mind).

- Dysautonomia, adrenal stress, or insufficiency (all of which can manifest as a hyper-alert appearance aka "deer in headlights").

- Disordered eating (lack of calories, good fats, and proteins can impact learning).[447]

All of these symptoms together or individually are often put under the umbrella of "brain fog" or simply diagnosed as ADD or ADHD. In my opinion, getting to the underlying cause of these behaviors and brain fog is vital, rather than just applying "name it, blame it, tame it" medicine. This is especially true for these cognitive issues, as medications conventionally used to manage ADD and ADHD may exacerbate the tics and anxiety seen with PANS/PANDAS.

Treatment

Overall, "brain fog" is treated as any other symptom in PANS/PANDAS with the three-pronged approach. We continue to treat any underlying infection, address inflammation, and provide immune support while reducing the actual symptom(s). For the last of these, it is important first to recognize what is behind the brain fog, such as sleep issues or anxiety, and treat that root cause.

Pharmaceutical Management

We sometimes consider prescription treatment for brain fog with Atomoxetine, a norepinephrine (noradrenaline) reuptake inhibitor approved for ADHD treatment.[448] In addition to its good track record of helping with concentration, the drug has anti-inflammatory properties as well, so it may be more beneficial than stimulant medications in treating children with PANS/PANDAS. Be aware that we first recommend an EKG to rule out a prolonged QT interval. Atomoxetine and a few other medications for attention and focus can further prolong this interval and may be contraindicated. Other non-stimulant medications, such as Viloxazine, have also been developed and may be worth consideration.

Other drugs to consider may include Guanfacine or long-acting Guanfacine (under the brand name of Intuniv), an alpha-blocker approved for treating ADD/ADHD. It may also be helpful in the treatment of anxiety, tics, and OCD.[449]

As with all medications, start low and titrate up weekly as tolerated. Initially, a child may experience sleepiness, so start on a weekend, and if there is no change within 2-3 days, consider dosing at night, as this can still be helpful. If a child develops a headache, stop immediately and consider an alternative.

Occasionally in children with PANS/PANDAS, we will trial stimulant medications if other pharmaceutical and natural interventions have been exhausted. We utilize stimulants last, as we have often seen an exacerbation of tics, OCD, and anxiety with these drugs. When prescribing stimulant medications, we recommend long-acting formulations, starting low and increasing slowly, as these are less likely to trigger these exacerbations.

Natural Interventions

Often equally or more effective than pharmaceuticals alone is *Bacopa monnieri,* a powerful antioxidant herb that reduces inflammation, boosts brain function, and helps reduce ADHD symptoms and anxiety.[450] Bacopa has been used for centuries in Ayurvedic medicine, either alone or in combination with other herbs, as a memory and learning enhancer, with good results.

We also employ multiple nutraceuticals, vitamins, and minerals to maintain normal and healthy brain function. These interventions may help to reduce inflammation in the brain, improve the child's ability to adapt to stressors and support the healthy and normal production of neurotransmitters. Because of the immense overlap of these with other common symptoms of PANS/PANDAS, all of these interventions have been included in other chapters. These include:

- Essential fatty acids/omegas

- Vitamin D

- Iron

- Zinc

- Magnesium

- B complex

Adjunct Treatment

Recommending adjunct therapy (perhaps Cognitive Behavioral Therapy, occupational therapy, neurofeedback, etc.) and emotional support or counseling to help both the child and family navigate the episodic course of these and all issues in PANS/PANDAS is crucial. These interventions are discussed in more depth in the Neurotherapy Chapter. With these issues in mind, we often write letters to schools on behalf of the families, offering helpful tips such as the following.

Organizational Support

- Preferential/assigned seating (up front and on the side, opposite the child's dominant ear)

- Use of assignment notebook planner/assignment sheets/online resources.

- Project break down, use of mnemonic devices, cues/prompts.

- Structured classroom: organize distraction-free study areas at work carrels.

Attention Supports

- Directions which are short, concise, and written if possible

- Positive feedback for what they are doing right

- Teacher/student/parent check-in by SPED to determine waxing/waning levels of attention and adjust/accommodate accordingly.

- Opportunities for breaks and movement when needed within the classroom.

Sensory Supports

- Accommodations for auditory overload or distraction: including the use of carpeting, tennis balls on chair legs, muting P.A. systems, and headphones.

- Accommodations for visual overload or distraction: muted colors in working areas, blinds to reduce sun glare, and the reduction of visual clutter

- Allow awareness of olfactory and tactile stressors.

Memory Supports

- Repetition and material review: teach in small bits of information that can be handled.

- Present new information in a meaningful context and not in a vacuum

- Help the child identify personal strengths and weaknesses in memorizing.

- Use a calculator, math facts sheets, digital tape recorder, smart pens, and lists.

Fine Motor Supports

- Extended time for all projects involving writing.

- Use of word processor, note taker, recording equipment, or graph paper.

- Shorten long assignments; allow the child to complete every other item.

- Use of oral responses, scribe, or recorder for tests.

General Supports

- Allow for early dismissal, late arrival, and excused absences without penalty.

- Provide alternative physical education (to accommodate clumsiness as well as anxiety).

- Allow fluid access to bathroom breaks without permission.

- Encourage rest periods, breaks, or fewer classes.

- Extended time on tests and assignments

One of the most important hallmarks of providing care for children with brain fog and PANS/PANDAS, in general, is to create and allow access to all accommodations without blaming or shaming while at the same time providing support that allows the child to succeed, rather than stagnate. This is a delicate balance that starts with understanding the nature of this neuropsychological illness, as well as compassion for the child and family going through this overwhelming relapsing and remitting disease course. Educating the child's community is the first step in achieving this goal.

SLEEP

As any parent can tell you, a child's sleep is, at best, tricky and, at worst, a disaster. Difficulty sleeping is quite common in childhood, so taken alone, abnormal sleep patterns or habits are not symptoms that would necessarily suggest PANS/PANDAS or Basal Ganglia Encephalitis. However, *abrupt* onset of sleeping problems, especially disinhibition during REM (Rapid Eye Movement) sleep or very restless sleep, is one of the most common somatic symptoms of PANS/PANDAS.

Studies show that children with PANS and PANDAS have trouble during REM sleep,[451] so even if the duration of your child's sleep falls within "normal," his sleep quality may not be adequate. Polysomnographic investigations show that 87% of children with Basal Ganglia Encephalitis have evidence of motor disinhibition during REM sleep. This results in excessive movement, moaning, or other forms of restless sleep. In addition, sleep loss amplifies preemptive responding in the amygdala,[452] significantly affecting those susceptible to anxiety. Conversely, sleep restoration may ameliorate anticipatory response and anxiety, strengthening the argument for adequate sleep in our children.

In addition, as we know through several studies, sleep is essential for immune restoration as well as natural detoxification.[453] If autoimmune encephalitis is at all on your list of differential diagnoses and the child is experiencing unrestful sleep, this symptom needs to be addressed early in treatment, as rest is essential to adequate immune, detoxification, and learning processes.

Treatment

Sleep Hygiene

The most basic of interventions families should implement is good sleep hygiene—essentially, setting the stage for ideal sleep conditions each night.

- Set a time to go to bed and a time to wake up. Be consistent!

- Make sure the bedroom is dark, quiet, cool, and comfortable

- Keep TVs, phones, computers, and all electronic devices out of the bedroom

- Limit the use of electronic devices of any kind before bedtime

- Ensure adequate exercise and daylight exposure

- Consume an anti-inflammatory diet consistent with circadian rhythm (i.e., protein in the morning and afternoon, simple carbohydrates later in the day).

Although these tips can be a handy guideline for a sleep hygiene plan, I have found the approach by Chris Winter, MD, the physician who penned *The Sleep Solution*, to be a great resource for parents and children to improve sleep.

Pharmaceuticals

Sleep can become so problematic that parents and practitioners are compelled to turn to prescription drugs as a solution. While there are currently no drugs approved to treat childhood insomnia, medications such as Mirtazapine (especially in children who also have seizures) or

Trazodone may be considered while under the care of a prescribing physician.[454] Exercise caution with the use of hypnotic sleep aids, such as Zolpidem, as psychosis and other side effects can occur.

As you know, inflammation is a hallmark of PANS/PANDAS, and concomitant allergies are quite common. The use of antihistamines, such as Diphenhydramine, may be beneficial for managing symptoms and encouraging sleep. However, at least 10% of children have paradoxical hyperactivity with these OTC medications, so consider other treatments if the child or a family member has already experienced this phenomenon.

Nutraceuticals

Melatonin is a hormone produced by the pineal gland that aids in the body's natural circadian rhythm.[455] Melatonin levels naturally rise in the evening and decrease prior to waking. A powerful antioxidant useful for cellular protection, melatonin may also help to regulate blood pressure, body temperature, cortisol levels, and immune function. A meta-analysis of nineteen studies shows that melatonin decreases sleep onset latency, increases total sleep time, and improves overall sleep quality.[456] Short-term melatonin use is safe for children, with minimal to no side effects. While more long-term studies are needed to assess the use of melatonin over extended periods of time, utilizing this natural intervention while other aspects of PANS/PANDAS are being addressed is a worthwhile treatment option.[457]

Some practitioners new to integrative medicine may be intimidated by botanical medicine, but herbs can be an incredible tool. Because of the minimal risks associated with these, consider utilizing *Passiflora incarnata* (passionflower), *Scutellaria lateriflora* (skullcap), *Matricaria chamomilla* (chamomile), *Valeriana officialis* (valerian), *Piper methysticum* (Kava Kava), *Lavandula angustifolia* (lavender), or

Withania somnifera (Ashwagandha). Many of these herbs and accompanying references are listed elsewhere in the guidebook. They can also help with anxiety, OCD, and tics, making them ideal for simplifying treatment plans and increasing compliance. Find preparations of these herbs that are non-alcoholic if possible (also known as glycerites), and consider diluting in water or juice to mask the herbal taste.

Nutraceuticals such as Gamma-Aminobutyric acid (GABA), L-theanine, and 5-hydroxytryptophan (5-HTP) can be useful for both sleep and anxiety. GABA is sometimes referred to as the "zen" neurotransmitter, so it is best used to minimize overexcitement, stabilize mood, and reduce stress.[458] It works in tandem with glutamate, the body's excitatory neurotransmitter, so finding a balance between the two can be an effective approach to brain health. L-theanine is a calmative amino acid that provides an essential element in the production of GABA, serotonin, and dopamine. It promotes general relaxation,[459] which can be an effective way to address brain health without directly altering neurotransmitter levels. 5-HTP is the immediate precursor in the production of serotonin. When serotonin levels are stable and optimal, symptoms of anxiety and depression are greatly reduced, and 5-HTP is then shunted into the pathway that produces melatonin—a great way to reduce anxiety *and* promote better sleep. In fact, a 2018 study showed that the combination of 5-HTP and GABA is more powerful than the administration of each nutrient alone, leading to longer sleep duration and improved sleep quality.[460] Do not use 5-HTP when a child is taking SSRIs, as this may increase the risk of serotonin syndrome.

Finally, magnesium. Magnesium is a calmative mineral that directly competes with excitatory calcium, promoting physical relaxation,[461] especially of the musculoskeletal system. Because of its high absorption through the skin, I often recommend nightly Epsom salt baths as part of a healthy sleep routine, encouraging one cup of magnesium sulfate together with one cup of alkalinizing baking soda per bath. For those who don't enjoy baths, magnesium glycinate can be dosed at dinnertime or before bed in a drink or gummy to address sleep. If constipation is also an issue in your child, magnesium citrate or magnesium oxide will provide laxative effects while also encouraging relaxation, as discussed in the Constipation chapter.

Other Factors

Keep in mind that microbial overgrowth—including yeast, parasites, bacteria, and viruses—should be investigated, as should underlying vitamin and mineral deficiencies, as these can all impact sleep as well. In addition to pharmaceuticals and nutraceuticals to treat these issues, as discussed in other chapters, appropriate diet management is essential to a good night's sleep and to treating nutritional deficiencies and microbial overgrowth that may impact sleep. Please refer to our Nutrition chapter for further dietary suggestions.

Parting Thoughts

In children with PANS and PANDAS, caregivers and practitioners must be aware that sleep issues can cause and affect many underlying health concerns, creating a hard-to-break cycle of pathology. Both as a cardinal symptom in PANS/PANDAS and its impact on quality of life, disordered sleep metabolism has a paramount impact on both diagnosis and care of a child in your practice.[462] By assessing and treating the whole child, addressing underlying causes, and supporting good sleep, a practitioner can help a child and family better deal with all of the issues associated with this devastating disease.

Constipation

Constipation is a common problem in children. It is neither indicative nor diagnostic of a PANS/PANDAS case. Still, it is frequent enough to consider treating, and I cannot stress enough the importance of addressing it immediately, prior to any nutraceutical or prolonged antimicrobial interventions.

If we consider the gastrointestinal tract and its importance in detoxification, constipation is a problem that must be addressed *before* multiple antimicrobial interventions can be entertained. Once we begin the process of eradicating infection, these microbes can cause side effects of "die-off," including symptoms indicative of Herxheimer reactions or healing crises. If the child's body is unable to detoxify the contents of the bowels because of constipation, these side effects are more severe and prolonged, adding to the inflammation that these children already experience.

Constipation is not just hard to pass or infrequent stools. It can include any one or several of the following:[463]

- Less than three bowel movements per week
- Less than one stool per day
- Bowel movements that are hard, dry, or difficult to pass
- Large stools that may clog the toilet

- Pain while having a bowel movement

- Abdominal pain, especially before bowel movements

- Irritable or agitated behavior, especially before bowel movements

- Traces of liquid or smears of stool in underwear

- Blood on the surface of hard stool

- Bloating, distention, especially before bowel movements

- Hands in pants, probing behaviors

- Urinary incontinence

In addition to issues with absorption and bioavailability of interventions, constipation is associated with autonomic dysfunction (heart rate variability) and anxiety in children with autism,[464] as well as ritualized behaviors and an increase in obsessive-compulsive behaviors.[465]

Constipation can have multiple causes, including but not limited to the following:

- Withholding: fear of the toilet, toilet training issues, desire to not stop play, being away from home, a vicious cycle of hard stools

- Diet: lack of fiber (fruits, veggies), lack of fluid, too much dairy

- Routine changes: stress, travel, weather

- Medications: antacids (with aluminum or calcium), antispasmodics, antidepressants, narcotics

- Metabolic issues: hypothyroidism, mitochondrial dysfunction

- Anatomic issues: Hirschsprung's, narrowing from obstruction, tumor

- Medical issues: IBD/IBS, Celiac disease, dysbiosis

Diagnosing Constipation

As always, history and physical examination are key, and asking for the details of stooling is essential. If a practitioner suspects constipation but cannot confirm it by exam, an abdominal x-ray may be indicated. Sometimes, lack of effective motility causes or exacerbates constipation, so utilizing an easy "motility test" for home testing is simple and informative. Recommend a meal with beets or have the child ingest a capsule of activated charcoal, then have parents monitor the time it takes to observe color change in stools. Typical timing is 12-24 hours, and any longer indicates constipation or slow motility. Further studies are often unnecessary but may include:

- Anorectal manometry

- Rectal biopsy

- Transit studies

- Stool microbiology, mycology, parasitology

Finally, blood tests that may be helpful include:

- CBC (to look for evidence of anemia of chronic disease)

- Thyroid panel

- Mitochondrial markers (carnitine, alanine: lysine ratio, fasting lactate, pyruvate)

- Minerals (RBC zinc and magnesium)

Treatment

Once constipation has been identified as part of the larger symptom picture, initial interventions focus on a high fiber diet, adequate fluid intake, exercise/movement, and routine changes surrounding stooling.[466]

- A high fiber diet includes beans, whole grains, fruits, and vegetables, often fourteen grams for every 1,000 calories. If a child does not have adequate fiber in their diet, you must begin slowly to reduce the amount of gas and bloating.[467]

- Water and naturally flavored water are ideal for achieving adequate fluid intake. Be sure to avoid cow's milk, as excess milk can contribute to constipation. Sodas and juice also count *against* the total daily intake of fluids, as these are pro-inflammatory and do not support detoxification.

- Adjust the child's routine to allow for adequate time for bowel movements (5-10 minutes after every meal), ideally in the comfort of their own homes. Additional praise and support (okay, *bribery*) can be important in encouraging good stooling rituals.

- Finally, good abdominal massage or professional visceral manipulation work may help a chronically constipated child by physically encouraging bowel movement.

In addition to each of the above common-sense interventions, I consider the following to further support gastrointestinal motility, tailored to each child's individual symptom picture. As with any intervention in children, starting low and increasing slowly for maximum benefit and minimum side effects is best.

- Oils: include liberally in cooking, such as olive and coconut oils, as well as essential fatty acids (fish oil) supplements.

- Vitamin C: this intervention should be considered carefully, as vitamin C can be an excellent cathartic but can also increase hyperactivity and agitation in susceptible children. Monitor for these symptoms closely. Note that vitamin C is a water-soluble vitamin; as such, any excess will be excreted through urination, so safety is not typically an issue.

- Magnesium: magnesium citrate or oxide is often the most effective form of magnesium when treating constipation. As an osmotic laxative,[468] it helps constipation and improves hyperactivity,[469] anxiety, tics/twitches as in TS,[470] and insomnia. Magnesium can be given orally but is also well absorbed via highly concentrated Epsom salt baths, which is ideal for those children who enjoy bath time or who have issues with oral supplements/medications.

- Aloe vera is an effective laxative and anti-inflammatory, although the aloe quality and certification are key. My rule of thumb is that if the aloe tastes too good, it is probably not pure aloe! Aloe is a succulent plant, and a stimulant laxative that aids digestion by stimulating the bowels[471] and decreasing inflammation.[472] The gel is odorless and safest for long-term use, while the juice or "latex" is yellow, bitter, and has stronger laxative properties, ideal for more short-term use.

- Senna: an herbal laxative used to increase motility, commonly found in teas.[473]

- Carnitine: an effective agent for mitochondrial support (necessary to alleviate other symptoms of PANS/PANDAS such as fatigue, brain fog, etc.). Carnitine insufficiency has been shown to exacerbate constipation.[474] Carnitine levels should be routinely monitored.

- Physical manipulation of the bowels via glycerin suppositories or enemas may be indicated if fecal impaction is suspected.

The Takeaway

When a child has constipation, treat this first. Constipation profoundly affects children with autoimmune encephalitis, PANS/PANDAS, and other chronic illnesses because it prevents healthy elimination of toxins, wreaking havoc on their already inflamed bodies.[475] Nutritious and detoxifying foods, adequate fluid intake, exercise, and healthy routines are essential for good stooling. As practitioners, we must look for underlying metabolic and mitochondrial problems while implementing these first-line interventions and use interventions as needed to get children pooping. Remember, it's not an apple a day that's important. It's a poop-a-day!

NEUROTHERAPY

As you now are well aware, the treatment of PANS/PANDAS is a three-pronged approach, focusing on antimicrobial treatment, immunomodulatory interventions, and symptom relief. Because we have so many pharmaceutical and herbal tools to relieve our patients' symptoms, it is easy to overlook the ways in which allied health professionals can complement our care. In my experience, however, a well-rounded care team providing physical, mental, and emotional support can make a huge impact on the trajectory of a child's healing and overall quality of life. Our clinic has found the most useful non-pharmacological approaches include Cognitive Behavioral Therapy (CBT), neurofeedback, mindfulness, and exercise.[476]

It is also important to remember therapy for the entire family. Siblings may well need therapy too. Understanding that genetic susceptibility can greatly contribute to a child's health picture, practitioners should remind families to identify signs and symptoms in other siblings without pathologizing each child's every move or mood change. Also, families should work with their therapists to avoid additional food-related OCD issues, especially for children with eating disorders.

Overall, for families and practitioners, it is essential to build a team. It takes a variety of interventions and a true village to care for our children and families.

Cognitive Behavioral Therapy

Cognitive Behavioral Therapy (CBT) is a form of psychotherapeutic treatment that helps children identify and alter the destructive thoughts that negatively impact their behaviors and emotions.[477] It is based on the belief that external events or triggers do not directly cause emotional behaviors but instead affect an individual's thought process, which determines the emotional and behavioral response. Therefore, by modifying their thoughts to be more positive and less self-sabotaging, the children undergoing CBT can minimize problematic behaviors such as OCD, anxiety, and rage.

Let's consider a simplified example that may help you better understand the benefits of CBT: the first time a child sleeps alone. A child may think there are monsters under the bed and thus, are scared. This can then lead to behaviors such as crying or trying to sleep with parents. A simple solution can be a night light. With the light on, the child can see there are no monsters, and the flawed belief is corrected. By "turning on the light," errant beliefs can be replaced with more logical and real evidence preventing corresponding behavioral issues.

This "turning on the light" correlates with the ABCs of CBT, a technique that helps challenge errant thinking.

- A is the adversity or activating event (going to sleep alone in a dark room).

- B is the belief about the event, including conscious and subconscious thoughts about the situation, others, or self (fear of monsters).

- C is the child's emotional and behavioral consequences (crying, tantrums).

By utilizing the ABC model, the therapist helps the child explore the relationship between B and C. By re-evaluating beliefs, healthier consequences and thoughts can be achieved whenever a triggering adverse or activating event occurs.[478]

In the context of Basal Ganglia Encephalitis, behaviors such as tics, ritualistic tendencies, OCD, separation anxiety, and eating disorders are both neurological and learned. Therefore in experienced hands,[479] CBT is beneficial for two reasons: it provides coping skills to help resolve symptoms more quickly and trains the brain to default to these coping skills by creating healthy routines. Although we have not found CBT to eliminate behaviors completely, it can be a very useful therapy for children and families to reduce their severity and frequency dramatically while also building a child's resilience. CBT is a well-researched therapy, typically utilized for at least four to seven months that this clinician has found invaluable as an adjunct to medical interventions.[480]

Neurofeedback

Put simply, neurofeedback therapy is the retraining a child's brainwave patterns to become more attentive or productive.[481] While a child engages in a neurofeedback activity, typically watching a movie or playing a video game, brainwaves in specific regions are recorded using EEG technology and analyzed in real-time. When these brain waves satisfy predetermined criteria for "healthy" brain activity, the patient receives positive feedback via the movie or video game. However, when the brainwaves fall below the threshold for healthy brain activity, the movie or video game will stop or become less engaging. The patient will have to say or mentally think "play" for the movie to continue. This process of rewarding certain patterns of brain activity via feedback retrains the brain to produce healthier brainwave patterns, resulting in improved behavioral functioning and attention.[482] Clinically, we see these healthier brain patterns manifest as decreased anxiety and OCD, with improvement in executive function deficits.[483] We generally find that around twenty neurofeedback sessions may be sufficient to ensure that new brainwave patterns take hold.[484]

Mindfulness

Mindfulness is a practice we like to recommend for the whole family, as it is useful for people of any age and ability level to ground and refocus. It encourages increasing one's awareness of thoughts, feelings, and self-sabotaging actions, and has well-documented positive impacts on mental and physical health.[485] Our children report improvements specifically with anxiety, eating disorders and OCD-related behaviors as well as improved sleep quality in family members.

Mindfulness works by helping people accept their experiences, including painful emotions, rather than avoiding them or engaging in other destructive coping behaviors. While mindfulness therapy is distinct from CBT, the two are often used together in treatment. Both help the individual gain perspective on their errant beliefs and how these thoughts may affect their behaviors in harmful ways.

The beauty of mindfulness is that it can include any technique that one finds calming and restorative, including movement (yoga, stretching), coloring, eating exercises, meditation, body scanning, and listening to music, among many others. The possibilities for utilizing mindfulness and tailoring activities for each family member are endless. As a daily practice of stress management[486], we encourage the life-long cultivation of this helpful skill.

Physical Activity

Another whole-family recommendation: exercise! Physical activity is connected to a myriad of mental health benefits in addition to the well-known physical benefits it imparts, including the reduction of anxiety, depression, and negative moods by boosting self-esteem and cognitive functioning.[487] A Harvard School of Public Health study showed a 26% reduction in the risk of depression with fifteen minutes per day of running or one hour per day of walking. This effect is correlated with neuronal growth, the release of endorphins, and decreased systemic inflammation. Interestingly, newer research suggests that exercise can alleviate the behavioral response by simulating similar physiological conditions experienced during anxiety and connecting this heightened physiological state to the enjoyable exercise experience instead of a fight or flight response. Over time, children may become less likely to panic when anxious in the future.[488] Exercise and any physical activity in children have been proven to have multiple positive effects on physical and psychological health and wellbeing. I cannot emphasize enough how big of a role this can play in supporting physical/emotional health and bonding for the entire family.

Case Studies

PANDAS/Autoimmunity: James

OCD and PANS/PANDAS: Dante

Multiple Infection PANS/PANDAS: Matt

Autism and Mycoplasma PANS/PANDAS: Rashad

Mycoplasma/OCD: Eva

Mitochondrial Dysfunction and Mycoplasma: Elijah

Multiple Infections, Vitamin Deficiency, and Mycotoxins: Sofia

Lyme, Multiple Co-Infections, and Basal Ganglia Encephalitis: Avery

PANDAS and Mold: Hannah

PANDAS, Mold, Babesia and Dysautonomia: Zevin

OCD/POTS: Kristen

Tics and Antioxidants: Caleb

PANDAS, Crohn's, and HDCs: Charlie

Autism and HDCs: Ty

PANS and COVID: Layla

PANDAS/Autoimmunity: James

Initial Presentation

- Sudden onset of regressive behavior, including tantrums and bouts of anger

- Emotional lability

- Extreme anxiety and new fears

- Hypersensitivity of his skin

- Ritualistic behaviors and obsessions

Past Medical History

- Severe constipation with rectal prolapse, encopresis for several years (previously treated with Miralax)

- Neurotypical until the onset of symptoms

Family Medical History

James' family medical history is significant for autoimmune diseases, including allergies, asthma, and thyroiditis. History of rheumatic fever in several grandparents and his father.

Dr. O'Hara's Notes

James is a 9-year-old child who presented to my office with recently diagnosed PANDAS. He is a sensitive but neurotypical child who previously had no other significant medical problems. As is pathognomonic in children with PANS/PANDAS, everything changed dramatically overnight while he and his family were on vacation. His mother insists he woke up as "a different kid" on August 25th. Suddenly, he was experiencing tantrums and intense anger and was emotionally labile.

In addition, his mother reports the abrupt onset of specific regressive behaviors, including a new fear of the dark and being alone. He would insist on being carried by his mother. He couldn't go anywhere without her, even to a different floor within their house. He developed an extreme sensitivity to cold and wet sensations and to the texture of his clothes. Within days came the onset of obsessive and ritualistic behaviors: he would only drink out of a certain cup, he would only walk in certain patterns, and his eating became very picky.

Mere days after the initial neurobehavioral change, James developed a choreiform movement of his head, rocking it back and forth. He would put his chin to his chest, then roll his head back and rock it three times until he cracked his neck. On August 28th, his parents took him to a walk-in clinic, where the doctor on duty visualized what he believed to be Strep throat. Unfortunately, the team was not able to perform a culture at that time because James was raging and trying to climb out of the window. Still, based on the history, the doctor suspected PANDAS and started him on a course of Amoxicillin-Clavulanate. James improved almost immediately after this antibiotic treatment, although he continued to experience severe constipation and picky eating, which his mom described as a "very bland and colorless" diet. In addition to these remaining symptoms, he continued to experience some OCD and handwriting deterioration, as well as more irritability and anxiety than usual.

In James' own words, prior to treatment with our clinic, he constantly felt very shaky, like he wanted to crawl out of his skin, and that he couldn't help himself. He wanted to be in the bathroom a lot because he was so anxious and felt the urge to pee all the time. He wanted to eat, but everything tasted like "starched shirts." He couldn't write or draw like he used to, and he was really tired. He had imaginary friends that he talked to because it made him feel safe. He always felt clumsy, stupid, afraid, and angry.

Signs and Symptoms

In addition to the symptoms that James' family discussed with me, an in-office physical examination revealed typical choreiform movements, the "piano-playing fingers." He had white spots on his nails but otherwise appeared healthy and normal.

Analysis

While PANDAS seemed very likely, I wanted to rule out a few other diagnoses that might exacerbate the neurological disturbance James was experiencing. Our team performed several tests, including Strep and Mycoplasma titers, which were normal. In addition to these, we investigated vitamin and mineral levels, Lyme western blot and co-infections, thyroid function (given his chronic constipation), and immune markers, including high sensitivity CRP, sedimentation rate, and thyroid antibodies, immunoglobulins, and Strep pneumococcal serotypes. All of these were normal. The only abnormalities we found were a low vitamin D of 24, a low RBC magnesium of 3.7, a low RBC zinc of 8.2, and a high ANA that was positive in a speckled pattern at 1:160. The ANA reflex panel was negative.

These are typical, essentially normal findings. Although we considered additional testing, the detailed history, and physical exam made us comfortable with our diagnosis, and the negative antibody titers were not unexpected. Based on his history of abrupt onset of multiple neuropsychiatric and somatic symptoms, his family history of rheumatic fever and autoimmune disease, and his rapid improvement with Amoxicillin-Clavulanate, we diagnosed him with PANDAS.

Treatment Plan

Because James had done so well with antibiotic treatment, we began prophylaxis with Azithromycin, as we wanted to avoid future Strep infections and recurrence of flares. We included a probiotic and *Saccharomyces boulardii* to keep yeast at bay and provide a prebiotic. To address his vitamin and mineral deficiencies, we prescribed vitamin D3 with K2 emulsion, zinc picolinate to support healthy immune function, and magnesium citrate to bowel tolerance. As magnesium citrate has laxative effects, we were able to wean James off of Miralax while also replenishing his mineral stores and calming his nervous system.

Tailoring his treatment to balance autoimmunity and provide mitochondrial support, we recommended Coenzyme Q10, Omega 3s in the form of fish oil, curcumin (an excellent anti-inflammatory), Cognitive Behavioral Therapy, and mindfulness exercises.

Progress Report

Several weeks after treatment began, James' mother reported that he was less irritable, more social, more cooperative, and had no tics or OCD. He was doing very well until months later, when he had what mom described as a "big flare" with increased irritability, OCD, and rigidity. A detailed intake revealed that he had lost several baby teeth and gained two canine teeth, causing him some inflammation and pain. This was a red flag: when children lose teeth or new teeth begin to erupt, the acute inflammation of the cranial nerves can trigger neurobehavioral flares. Anti-inflammatories like Ibuprofen can be very helpful to soothe the pain and decrease neuropsychiatric involvement.

Later, his mother reported that James experienced another significant flare when his sister developed Strep throat. At that time, he did not show any signs or symptoms of Strep throat, but his Strep culture was positive. Much like the acute stress of active dentition, Strep infections in other family members or close members of the child's community can trigger neuroinflammation. Many children have behavioral flares when their siblings are diagnosed with Strep or other infectious diseases. Thus, it is important to check the child for Strep whenever there are behavioral flares and/or a close contact is diagnosed, despite a lack of throat or Strep-related symptoms. To address this, we changed his antibiotics, prescribed a short round of additional anti-inflammatories, and prescribed prophylactic antimicrobials to his sister for a time to prevent her from contracting Strep in the near future.

With these treatments, James told us that he felt calmer. He didn't need to talk to himself as much to calm down. He still felt anxious but felt he could manage it and work through it. He didn't feel the need to write things over and over. He could play in gym class or with his friends again without feeling like he was going to fall. His handwriting normalized, and thankfully, he felt more like himself.

Summary

James is a classic example of Strep-induced PANDAS or Basal Ganglia Encephalitis, given the abrupt onset, the initial findings of Strep pharyngitis on the exam, choreiform movements, a family history of rheumatic fever, and his improvement with antibiotics and natural immunotherapy. His case also illustrates some other triggers that can induce flares, such as teething and infections in siblings or other close contacts that need to be identified and appropriately treated.

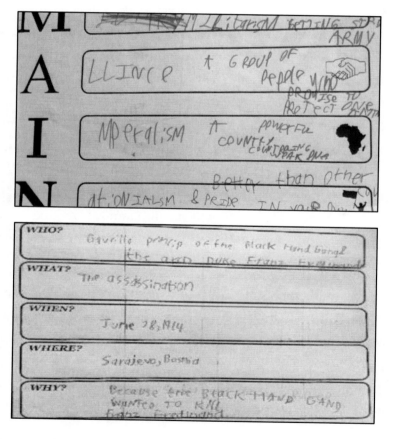

Handwriting Changes During PANDAS Flare and After Appropriate Management

OCD AND PANS/PANDAS: DANTE

Initial Presentation

- Verbal tics

- Ritualistic OCD behavior

- Hyperactivity

- Uncontrolled agitation and aggression

Past Medical History

- Mild form of autism

- Recurring sore throat

- Multiple previous positive Strep cultures, including one taken two months prior to the onset of symptoms

While Dante had been previously diagnosed with autism, he was quite high-functioning and did not experience any medical challenges associated with his condition. However, his history of frequent sore throats and the abrupt onset of his symptoms were significant red flags for PANDAS and neuroinflammation.

Family Medical History

No significant family medical history was noted.

Dr. O'Hara's Notes

Dante, an 8-year-old with a mild form of autism and a history of recurrent sore throats, had a sudden change in behavior about six months before presenting to my office. He developed verbal tics and ritualistic OCD behaviors, particularly regarding doors. He became hyperactive and began experiencing uncontrolled agitation and aggression, initially toward his brothers but later toward others as well. In the months since the onset of these behavioral changes, he had been put on multiple antipsychotic medications and even psychiatrically hospitalized, to no avail. His parents reported that his behavior was "beyond their control," and they were fearful that his condition would deteriorate further.

Signs and Symptoms

Dante exhibited piano-playing fingers (choreiform movements of hands), but the physical examination was otherwise unremarkable.

Analysis

In any child with a sudden onset of neuropsychiatric symptoms, Basal Ganglia Encephalitis must be considered, in addition to other diagnoses in the differential. You must rule out trauma, illicit drug or medication overdoses, abuse, meningitis/encephalitis, and other pertinent conclusions as described earlier in this guidebook. PANS or PANDAS was immediately suspected because of the sudden onset of agitation, OCD, ritualistic behaviors, and tics. Though Dante had a history of sore throats, he had no signs or symptoms of the pharyngeal disease at the time of presentation, and as noted below, Strep culture was negative. However, given the history and abrupt onset, as well as the choreiform movements on physical exam, we felt that it was prudent to consider a trial of antibiotics, as PANDAS was most likely.

Test Results

- Strep culture was negative

- All blood work was negative, including Mycoplasma and Strep titers (ASO and antiDNaseB Ab) and Lyme testing.

- RBC zinc and magnesium were low

Initial Treatment Plan

Dante was immediately prescribed Amoxicillin to address the possibility of PANDAS. We added probiotics and prebiotics to restore microbiome balance, plus zinc and magnesium to address his low levels. Additionally, he was put on activated charcoal for alkalinization and to treat any die-off or Herxheimers reactions, as can be seen in early treatment with antibiotics or other antimicrobials.

With one course of Amoxicillin, Dante got better. Immunotherapy, in the form of a short burst of steroids, was then added, and Dante's symptoms resolved completely. As we did not want to continue long-term Amoxicillin, he was prescribed antibiotic prophylaxis with Azithromycin. He remained symptom-free on this regimen for the remainder of the year.

Progress Report

Sometime after he found success with the initial treatment, Dante's family relocated to another state, lost touch with our practice, and stopped the preventive Azithromycin. Over the following few months, Dante's behaviors became episodically worse. His mother could not correlate any triggers with these episodes, which included additional ritualistic behaviors, anxiety, and significant agitation. He was put on Aripiprazole by his psychiatrist, which initially seemed to help.

However, the Apripiprazole was eventually no longer effective, and he was again hospitalized for aggression, agitation, and anxiety. His more recent symptoms also included auditory sensitivities and severe insomnia, motivated by searching the internet. CSF analysis, CT scans, EEG, and other testing were all negative.

Following Up

Out of ideas and resources, the family traveled back to our office. We ran a full panel of tests, including Strep, Mycoplasma, and Lyme titers, appropriate vitamin and mineral levels, and organic acid evaluation. His ASO, antiDNaseB antibody, Lyme, and co-infections were negative, as were his ANA and other inflammatory markers. However, his acute Mycoplasma antibodies were elevated. He had a very high Mycoplasma IgM and immunofluorescent assay (IFA). In addition, he had low vitamin D, magnesium, and zinc, which is quite common in our patients with PANS/PANDAS or other chronic illnesses.

Dante was prescribed Azithromycin to address the Mycoplasma infection, which yielded immediate improvement. We again attempted steroid therapy to assist with inflammation, but he, unfortunately, had increased agitation from this, so we shifted our approach. When a child responds negatively to steroid therapy, other germ overgrowths, particularly yeast, should be suspected. His organic acid test confirmed yeast, and he was therefore again put on a probiotic and prebiotic to nourish healthy flora. Healthy dietary choices were also discussed and proved helpful.

In addition to the continued course of Azithromycin, with the now more severe symptoms, his immunologist received approval for IVIG.

Before IVIG, Dante reported having extreme anxiety, which caused severe sensory-seeking OCD behaviors on the internet. He would stay up at night, excessively talking, running up and down the stairs, saying he wanted to sleep but could not. He would act impulsively and develop imaginary friends to combat his anxiety. After the IVIG was started, Dante became calmer, redirectable, less confrontational, and less threatening. He was better connected and engaged. Although his anxiety was still present, he was able to manage and work through it independently. He reported that "he felt more like himself."

Summary

Dante provides us with an initial example of the abrupt onset of symptoms with Basal Ganglia Encephalitis. At first, this was most likely caused by Strep and PANDAS, given his chronic and recent history of throat infections and his improvement with Amoxicillin and immunotherapy. It also provides us with an example of a need for ongoing prevention, either with Azithromycin, Penicillin, or herbal interventions (as we will see in other cases). The subsequent flares can be much worse when prophylactic antibiotics or antimicrobials are not maintained. These flares can be episodic and not easily correlated with recent infections. In Dante's case, he re-presented with PANS and Mycoplasma infection, requiring further antibiotics and immunotherapy, this time with IVIG. Fortunately, with appropriate management, he improved and was maintained until puberty on preventive antimicrobials.

Multiple Infection PANS/PANDAS: Matt

Initial Presentation

- Seizure-like tics
- Mild OCD
- Anxiety
- Regression in school

Past Medical History

- Minor sensory processing issues in childhood
- Bitten by Lyme-positive tick
- Strep throat
- Upper respiratory viral illness

Dr. O'Hara's Notes

Matt presented to our office as a 10-year-old boy with a sudden onset of seizure-like tics. He would be sitting, doing his homework, then suddenly end up looking like he was seizing on the floor. His tics were extremely violent and progressive. He also developed some mild OCD, anxiety (worries about health, separation from mom when he had been previously very independent), and a regression in his attention and ability to complete assignments at school.

Matt had previously been a healthy child, born by normal spontaneous vaginal delivery. He was breastfed, had a healthy environment, and ate an organic, gluten-free, casein-free diet. He had some sensory processing issues, but he was otherwise a neurotypical child before the onset of these tics. His recent past medical history included a viral illness with upper respiratory symptoms, Strep throat, and being bitten by a Lyme-positive tick the week before the onset of these neurological symptoms.

Physical Examination and Laboratory Evaluation

Physical examination was within normal limits, and all of the blood work we ordered was normal. Although he initially had negative Strep titers, a repeat test six weeks later showed elevated ASO and antiDNaseB antibodies. He also had an elevated ANA, low vitamin D, low zinc, and positive Lyme western blot at that time.

Treatment

Matt was treated for three months with antibiotics, then switched to an herbal rotation for maintenance. During those initial three months, he was also treated with HDCs (helminth therapy–see HDCs chapter for more information), zinc, vitamin D3, and essential fatty acids.

After the initial round of treatment, his tics resolved, but he was left with some amount of OCD and anxiety, as well as a 504 plan for school. He was resigned to the idea that "this was just who he was." He continued to progress with an episodic course of behavioral and executive function challenges for the following six or seven years.

Follow Up

At age 17, Matt returned to us. We discovered that he had a series of blanching stretch marks that did not follow dermal lines (striae), which suggested Bartonella. Testing proved positive for Bartonella, and he was started on Azithromycin, Rifampin, and Artemisinin, as well as other antimicrobial herbs. His tics became much, much worse as treatment began, similar to what he had experienced at age ten. We believe that he was experiencing a Herxheimer reaction, worsening symptoms before potential improvement. The tics remained severe for several weeks, but they resolved after about six weeks of treatment. In addition, and quite remarkably to his family, his anxiety, OCD, and need for a 504 resolved as well.

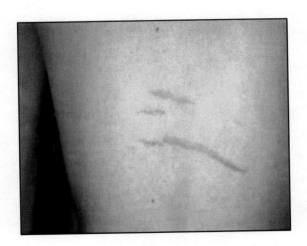

Bartonella Striae

In retrospect, we believe he had had Bartonella for many years, perhaps even from the initial presentation, but it had not been fully or adequately treated. Upon treating it, the tics came back initially (as with any healing crisis), but they then resolved with full treatment—as did his OCD, anxiety, attention, and learning differences.

He did well again for the next three years, but at age 20, he was significantly exposed to mold in his apartment. When he returned to us, his mycotoxin levels, particularly ochratoxin, were very high. Lyme testing at that time was entirely negative. Because of this mold exposure, he developed brain fog and a resurgence of some amount of OCD and anxiety. He was put on a binder for the ochratoxin and higher doses of essential fatty acids. The apartment was remediated. After a three-month course with binders and the apartment remediation, Matt's OCD and brain fog again resolved.

Summary

Matt's story illustrates the multifactorial nature of PANS/PANDAS and how a susceptible individual may be afflicted over time: first with Strep, possibly a virus and Lyme, with Bartonella, and then with mold. In susceptible individuals, all of these triggers need to be assessed and monitored. The episodic course of PANS/PANDAS, the waxing and waning, must be analyzed and treated as symptoms come and go and may progress. Matt is now thriving, getting a graduate degree, and living a healthy and full life. Only with ongoing education and vigilance can a child with Basal Ganglia Encephalitis reach their fullest potential.

Autism and Mycoplasma PANS/PANDAS: Rashad

Initial Presentation

- Movement disorder/Tics

- Rash

- Hallucinations

- Loss of academic ability

Past Medical History

- Failure to thrive in infancy

- Autism Spectrum Disorder (high-functioning, diagnosed around age four)

Dr. O'Hara's Notes

Rashad was a very happy, sweet little boy, and his family reports that he was always very sensitive to things. He had difficulty with sleep as a baby; he always needed to be moving in a swing, a car, etc. He was diagnosed with failure to thrive at two months, and a G tube was placed.

Although he had to be fed more often, he was concurrently breastfed and started to improve. When he was weaning from breastfeeding at twelve months, he began to lose weight, so his mother continued breastfeeding until he was two years old.

Rashad was still easily overwhelmed and would cry with loud noises, but at three years old, he went to preschool. He did well there, as there was a good amount of structure at that school, but at four years old, he was placed in a play-based preschool and was always on the perimeter.

He was diagnosed with high-functioning autism at that time, between the ages of four and five. He had some fine motor, gross motor, and sensory processing disorders, and he was supported with occupational therapy, physical therapy, and some behavioral therapy. Consequently, he became very interested in the arts. He was transferred to a different school in the third grade and was doing very well. He had friends at this school, was voted class president in fifth grade, and had completely caught up on his school work. He went to sleep away camp, and his family reported that "everything was going great."

At 11 years old, however, on October 18th, he got sick. His breathing was labored, and when he went to a pediatrician, his family was told he "had a virus." On October 25th, he developed a rash. By October 27th the rash progressed from his hands to his face and neck. He went to urgent care, who diagnosed him with allergies. The rash continued to spread, and on the night of October 30th, his respiratory symptoms worsened, and Rashad started having abnormal movements. He returned to urgent care, and they told him it was a tic. They believed he had pneumonia and prescribed a brief course of Azithromycin, cough suppressant, and Albuterol.

Despite treatment, Rashad's tics worsened, so he was ordered to have an EEG, CT scan, lumbar puncture, and to see a neurologist. He was diagnosed with a complex movement disorder. He returned to school, where the school psychologist actually told the mom that he should be tested for PANS and PANDAS.

By November 8th, OCD behaviors emerged, and he developed a headache that would not go away. He went to the emergency room, but nothing seemed to help. He was admitted to neurology, who performed an MRI and an overnight EEG. He was diagnosed again with a stereotypic movement disorder, and all other testing was negative. He continued to have other symptoms, including neuropathy, and was then readmitted and diagnosed with a conversion disorder. For that, he was prescribed an SSRI, Citalopram.

Rashad's rash continued to come and go. He was having hallucinations. He had lost academic skills, particularly in math. Eventually, other blood testing was performed. Mycoplasma was significantly positive. His doctors were hesitant to treat the Mycoplasma because he had already been treated with Azithromycin, but Rashad admitted at that time that he did not take the antibiotic and had been hiding the pills. It was then that he and his family came to see us.

Analysis

Rashad's medical history included the onset of rash, tics, OCD behavior, a history of possible viral infections, a diagnosis of conversion disorder, and a present and prolonged battle with Mycoplasma. Combined with physical exam findings that included nasal and sinus congestion, abdominal bloating, keratosis, and choreiform movements, we preliminarily diagnosed him with constipation, possible allergies, and PANS triggered by Mycoplasma.

Treatment

We started him on Azithromycin, and the tics and conversion symptoms improved. At that same time, his other physicians began to titrate the Citalopram. He also had allergic rhinitis, significant bloating, constipation, and other bowel symptoms, which we began to address.

We decided to increase Rashad's dose of Azithromycin. We created a supportive plan consisting of the following: a probiotic to maintain microbial balance, xylitol to break up his nasal congestion, increased hemp oil, the adaptogenic herb Ashwagandha to regulate his stress, and essential fatty acids, and additional anti-inflammatories to help with the chronic Mycoplasma. He was given dietary recommendations to reduce inflammation, and an acute viral protocol was discussed with the family in case he had any further viral infections.

Follow-Up

At the time of his next follow-up, it was found that his Mycoplasma infection had not resolved. However, he had negative Strep titers and negative inflammatory markers and weaned off the Citalopram successfully. He was eating well. He still had some bloating, but his brain function had improved dramatically, and he was able to attend school. He reported that he was falling asleep more easily, and his hallucinations had gone away completely. In general, he just felt better.

Magnesium and Epsom salt baths were added for constipation. He continued on the Azithromycin to treat Mycoplasma. Rashad had additional waxing and waning of symptoms after a tooth extraction and during periodic viral infections. With each, we increased and modified his antimicrobials, anti-inflammatories, and metabolic and detoxification support. He continues to do well with dietary interventions, exercise, improved sleep hygiene, continued magnesium and aloe to prevent constipation, and a rotation of herbal antimicrobials, antioxidants, and minerals supplementation. Rashad's case illustrates that even with significant psychiatric symptoms, appropriate diagnosis and treatment, including that of PANS, can lead to improvements.

MYCOPLASMA/OCD:
EVA

[Note: Eva's sibling is Elijah, who is featured in the next case study on mitochondrial dysfunction and Mycoplasma.]

Initial Presentation

- Sudden onset of anxiety

- OCD in the form of cleaning and hoarding

Past Medical History

- Previously healthy child

Dr. O'Hara's Notes

Previously healthy, Eva developed a sudden onset of anxiety and OCD, mainly in the form of hoarding and cleaning. She was hoarding everything in her bedroom and then began excessively cleaning. She had marked sadness and was constantly crying. After taking an extensive history, we learned that her grandfather had recently been hospitalized with pneumonia.

Physical Exam

Eva exhibited "piano-playing fingers" or choreiform movements when she came into the office, but her physical exam was otherwise unremarkable.

Analysis

Because Eva's younger sibling was diagnosed with mitochondrial dysfunction, it was certainly included in our testing. Given her grandfather's recent hospitalization for pneumonia, we also wanted to investigate an infectious cause of the OCD and choreiform movements and tested Eva for Mycoplasma as well as other infections.

Testing

Like her brother, Eva's testing was positive–both IgM and immunofluorescence assay (IFA) for Mycoplasma. We also found that Eva had minor mitochondrial abnormalities, including a slight elevation in liver enzyme AST (sometimes a more subtle sign of mitochondrial dysfunction), a high creatine kinase, and low carnitine.

Treatment

Eva showed improvement on Azithromycin, with only slight OCD remaining. Because her grandfather's sputum culture proved sensitive to tetracyclines, we prescribed a short round of Minocycline, eradicating her symptoms. To address her minor mitochondrial abnormalities, we provided glutathione support in the form of n-acetyl cysteine and CoQ10, and carnitine. As a preventive treatment, she continued on antimicrobials to prevent exacerbations of OCD and anxiety caused by infections.

Follow-Up

At her one-month follow-up, Eva was much calmer, reporting that she was happier and had not experienced the need to obsessively clean or hoard since she began the treatment protocol. She continues on mitochondrial support and sees our staff on an as-needed basis.

Mitochondrial Dysfunction and Mycoplasma:
Elijah

Initial Presentation

- Hypotonia
- Chronic diarrhea
- Fatigue
- Poor sleep

Past Medical History

- Hypotonia and hyperbilirubinemia with jaundice at birth
- Developmental delays in early childhood
- OXPHOS, a Complex I mitochondrial disorder

Dr. O'Hara's Notes

Elijah was born with neonatal jaundice, hyperbilirubinemia, and difficulty feeding caused by an inefficient latch. Subsequently, he had low muscle tone, had several developmental delays, and was experiencing chronic diarrhea, excessive fatigue, and poor sleep when he first presented to our office. After extensive history taking and testing, Elijah was diagnosed with OXPHOS, a Complex 1 mitochondrial disorder that causes dysfunction in the oxidative phosphorylation process.

Testing

At his initial presentation, Elijah's blood work revealed that he had a high AST, high lactate, high pyruvate, high ammonia, high alanine, low carnitine, and high MMA or methylmalonic acid, which is concomitant with a low intracellular B12 level, all consistent with a mitochondrial disorder.

Treatment

Elijah was treated with carnitine, a B vitamin complex, and additional B12, CoQ10, folinic acid, and essential fatty acids and was followed by a neurologist with expertise in mitochondrial disease and dysfunction.

Follow Up

Elijah saw great success for several years after we, together with his mitochondrial disease specialists, began treating his mitochondrial disorder. However, at age 11, he had a sudden onset of anxiety. At the same time, his healthy sibling, Eva, had a similar sudden onset of anxiety and OCD; her story can be found in the previous chapter.

When he presented to our office, Elijah was experiencing a marked regression. He was moodier in school, his attention span was very short, and he was greatly fatigued. We took another extensive history and learned that his grandfather had just been hospitalized with pneumonia. Elijah's testing at that time was positive for Mycoplasma, both IgM and IFA (immunofluorescent assay), and his grandfather tested positive for *Mycoplasma pneumoniae*.

Treatment consisted of an initial round of Azithromycin, and Elijah experienced marked improvements on this antibiotic, though not a full remission of symptoms. His grandfather still showed persistent symptoms of pneumonia with a cough, and his cultures returned, showing sensitivity to tetracyclines. Thus, Elijah was started on Minocycline at that time. This helped to improve his school performance and relieved the obsessive writing of which he had been complaining.

To further support what we suspected was a taxed mitochondrial load, Elijah was also placed on additional CoQ10 and n-acetyl cysteine, with added anti-inflammatory and mitochondrial support. Because his family was uncomfortable with prophylactic antibiotics, we instead recommended herbal antimicrobials, including a rotation of goldenseal, colloidal silver, and oil of oregano.

Currently, Elijah continues on a prophylactic antimicrobial rotation of herbs and ongoing mitochondrial support, and we see him on an as-needed basis.

Multiple Infections, Vitamin Deficiency, and Mycotoxins: Sofia

Initial Presentation

- Severe motor tics appearing as body convulsions
- Severe verbal tics, including coprolalia

Past Medical History

- Frequent sinus infections
- Persistent hiccups
- Constant sniffling and throat clearing

Dr. O'Hara's Notes

Sofia came to us as a seven-year-old with severe tics. She had a history of multiple sinus infections in early childhood, and at age four, she developed a persistent hiccup noise, constant sniffing, and throat clearing. Her mother felt that this was related to seasonal allergies, post nasal drip, and congestion from her extensive history of sinus and upper respiratory infections, and it waxed and waned over the years.

By age five, Sofia developed severe tics that looked like body convulsions. To her family, these tics looked like seizures, though they were not, and EEGs were always normal. Nothing seemed to help. At age six, her mother began to notice a marked red anal ring, and she reports that Sofia developed some urinary symptoms and mouth ulcers at that time. Shortly before she presented to our office, she developed severe vocal tics, including cursing and a classic Coxsackie rash.

Physical Exam and Testing

The physical exam confirmed a red anal ring and Coxsackie rash on the soles of her feet but was otherwise unremarkable. We decided to run extensive testing, including testing Sofia's parents. We found that Sofia had a very low level of vitamin A, acute IgM viral titers for Coxsackie A and B, and an elevated cam kinase level of 186, indicating that she may have had Strep infections leading to PANDAS. Her mother and father had high Strep and Mycoplasma titers, although Sofia's were normal.

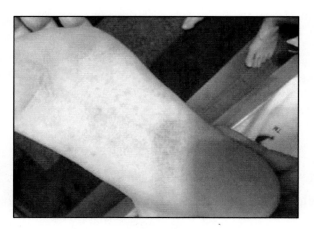

Coxsackie
(hand-foot-and-mouth disease)

Treatment

Her parents were prescribed Azithromycin by their practitioners, as was Sofia, and probiotic supplementation to address infections. For Sofia, we recommended a preparation of buffered n-acetyl cysteine because this often helps OCD and tics, as described in earlier chapters. We also recommended methylfolate because of a baseline MTHFR c677 defect we found in her bloodwork, in addition to its calming benefits.

Follow Up

Sofia and her family reported improvement in her tics and some decrease in her anxiety. Because her symptoms did not resolve fully, and because of the significantly low values we had found on initial blood work, we began a trial of high-dose vitamin A, as this has been reported to help with measles and other forms of viral encephalitis as outlined in earlier chapters, and the results were quite remarkable.

With the inclusion of vitamin A, Sofia's mother reported a noticeable decrease in Sofia's tics. Although she had been inundated with illnesses circulating at her school, she was not experiencing a worsening of her tics and only experienced minor facial and upper body tics (but no verbal tics anymore). She did note that when Sofia was exposed to a viral trigger, she developed a minor tic which manifested as a few quick vocal yelps, but otherwise, she had been doing very well.

Because of her significant progress, we recommended that she maintain a weekly protocol of vitamin A (while continuously monitoring her blood levels), N-acetyl cysteine, fish oil, methylfolate, lysine (an amino acid that has excellent antiviral properties), vitamin D3 for low vitamin D levels, an herbal rotation for prophylaxis, aloe for its anti-inflammatory action and effects on bowel health, Epsom salt baths, and probiotics. She continued to do well with minimally appreciable tics.

A few months later, Sofia returned to our office after her parents noticed a flood in their basement, and she had regressed. At that time, she had no improvement with antivirals, so we began extensive testing. Sofia was found to have high urine mycotoxins levels and evidence of CIRS. Multiple species of mold were found in the basement. We immediately recommended mold remediation, treatment with binders, and a biofilm protocol with a rotation of herbs, including oil of oregano, grapefruit seed extract, caprylic acid, and goldenseal. All of her symptoms resolved with this treatment. Although she still has occasional and very mild tics with infections, Sofia has had full remission of her symptoms.

Lyme, Multiple Co-Infections, and Basal Ganglia Encephalitis: Avery

Initial Presentation

- Abrupt onset of OCD behaviors

- Severe anxiety

Past Medical History

- Previous providers had suggested the onset of psychosis

Avery had had bronchitis as well as several instances of positive Strep cultures in her youth. She had been diagnosed with Lyme disease twice and was treated with two weeks of antibiotic therapy each time. She had a history of chronic ear infections treated with multiple antibiotics.

Dr. O'Hara's Notes

Avery was a 16-year-old star athlete when she first came to our office. She was a softball player being recruited by many colleges and a straight-A student. She was social and active until she experienced a sudden change in behavior that caused an acute onset of numerous paralyzing OCD behaviors. Mom can remember the day everything changed, March 4th. She started walking backward and sideways and along the edges of stairs. She constantly felt compelled to do a quick spin in an odd, quirky manner. She developed sensory issues, resisted wearing clothes, wore socks bunched up, and began to look very disheveled. She would not shower, and she stopped using the bathroom. She would not leave the family room and would defecate and urinate on a small section of the floor there. Her world grew progressively smaller. Her medical team at the time felt that this was psychiatric, perhaps the acute onset of psychosis, but her parents consulted us and others to rule out other causes and treatment of her disease state. When we dug deeper into her history, we were immediately concerned about Basal Ganglia Encephalitis.

Signs and Symptoms

Upon physical exam, Avery had one blanching stretch mark on her knee. All other findings were unremarkable.

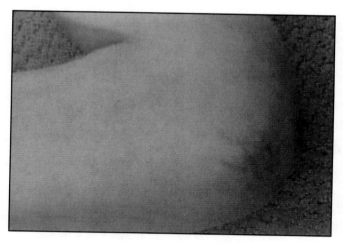

Bartonella Striae on Knee

Analysis

Because of the extensive history of recurring infections (Strep, Lyme, possible Mycoplasma or viral bronchitis, and striae consistent with Bartonella) and probable short-term and incomplete antibiotic treatment, our team evaluated her for each of these suspected infections and began a comprehensive treatment plan.

Test Results

Avery's initial test results showed a normal CBC, liver and kidney function, mitochondrial markers, sedimentation rate, thyroid function, and vitamin and mineral levels. She also had negative ANA, Strep titers, viral titers, and thyroid antibodies. Her MTHFR studies revealed that she was compound heterozygous, and on organic acid testing, she had multiple high yeast markers, including arabinitol. She had low IgG, IgG subclasses, and IgA subclasses. She had very high antibodies to multiple inflammatory markers in blood and cerebrospinal fluid testing. She also had Lyme results from a local hospital lab that showed multiple positive and significant IgM bands. Finally, Avery was positive for Bartonella through FISH, PCR, and western blot testing.

Initial Treatment Plan

Because Avery showed signs of yeast, Bartonella, and Lyme, she was immediately started on a protocol of antimicrobials, immunotherapy, anti-inflammatory interventions, and restorative nutrients. This included an anti-inflammatory diet and supplementation of aloe, probiotics, and prebiotics to support normal gastrointestinal flora.

We prescribed ongoing curcumin, quercetin, and Ibuprofen for acute flares to decrease inflammation. She was put on methyltetrahydrofolate to support healthy methylation and her MTHFR genetic defects. We further supported detoxification with milk thistle and naturally detoxifying interventions such as Epsom salt baths and activated charcoal capsules. She began an herbal rotation for yeast, which included oil of oregano, a pine bark extract called Taiga, olive leaf extract, and grapefruit seed extract.

In addition to her herbal rotation, Avery needed aggressive antibiotic therapy to treat Bartonella and Lyme diseases. She was put on Azithromycin, Cefdinir, and Bactrim to accomplish this.

Progress Report

After three months of this very aggressive treatment plan, she improved. We attempted to wean her from these medications, but her anxiety and other symptoms only worsened. Her family then trialed multiple SSRIs, antipsychotics, and anxiolytics. The methyltetrahydrofolate was switched to a prescription form, and her antibiotics were changed to Minocycline instead of Azithromycin, Rifampin instead of Bactrim, and Augmentin instead of Cefdinir. She continued on a rotation of anti-inflammatories, including curcumin and resveratrol, and was put on additional antioxidants and metabolic support. She had a team of physicians and other healthcare providers caring for her and supporting her and her family.

Unfortunately, she continued to worsen and developed an eating disorder as part of her worsening disease. Together with her infectious disease specialist and other doctors, she was placed on IV Ceftriaxone and Actigall to prevent any gallbladder disease. Because she also had evidence of chronic inflammatory demyelinating polyneuropathy—a peripheral neuropathy that is sometimes seen in children with PANS, PANDAS, and Lyme—she was approved by her insurance for IVIG. Thankfully, she started to improve with this treatment. She was able to dress, use the toilet, eat on her own, and get out of the house (although still unshowered).

Testing then showed cerebrospinal fluid positive for Lyme and more markedly positive peripheral Bartonella testing at this point, which is often the case. Initially, Bartonella testing can be negative or minimally positive until treatment is started. We feel that this means that any indication that Bartonella might be present should lead a practitioner to treat it, even without significantly positive testing. In addition, when one co-infection is found, others may become positive, so a vigilant approach is warranted. Avery also tested positive for Babesia during this time, and her immunologist began Atovaquone-Proguanil.

After multiple interventions, consultations with multiple specialists, and continuing to address the multisystem nature of her disease, Avery is finally improving. She cares about her hygiene. She was able to go back to school and is currently applying to colleges and continues to thrive.

Summary

This case represents a very complicated and severe onset of disease that can be seen in Basal Ganglia Encephalitis, especially when multiple infectious agents, in addition to Strep, are at play. For Avery, this included Lyme and co-infections of Bartonella and Babesia, though all psychiatric and medical diagnoses were considered and ruled out by testing and treatment trials. The keys to her success include a multidimensional and multi-specialty approach, with the constant support of the entire family.

PANDAS AND MOLD:
HANNAH

Initial Presentation

- Anxiety

- Difficulty with transition

- Anger/rage

- Severe mood swings

- Headaches

- Itchiness across body

Past Medical History

- Herpes simplex

- Conjunctivitis

- Constipation

Hannah was a happy, easy-going six-year-old girl with a history of childhood illnesses, including herpes cold sores, conjunctivitis, and occasional ear and respiratory infections. At age five, she enrolled in school and subsequently developed a sore throat and fever, which resolved on its own within a few days. Shortly after this illness, her behavioral issues began.

Family Medical History

Hannah's family history is significant for autoimmune disorders on both sides. Her mother has psoriasis, her father's family has thyroiditis and depression, and her maternal grandmother has fibromyalgia.

Dr. O'Hara's Notes

Hannah, a six-year-old child, presented to our office with a sudden onset of anger/rage and other behavioral changes. Her parents first noticed a change in her normally pleasant and calm personality at a horse riding lesson when she refused to participate. A few days later, Hannah complained about being sensitive to loud noises and began having issues with her friends at school "being mean" to her, although her teacher reported that *she* was being mean to and acting angry with them. At night, she was very angry about being told to go to bed, so much so that she kicked her bedroom wall for an hour in protest. She had never acted so aggressively in the past.

Shortly after, her anger and aggression began to develop, and anxiety soon followed. Hannah found being at school very difficult. Rages became a daily occurrence, particularly around transitions between lessons or locations, and the teaching staff would request for her to return home early. She struggled at bedtime, requiring hours of reading, singing, and consoling to relax enough to fall asleep.

Fortunately, Hannah's school staff was well-versed in the neurobehavioral symptoms of infectious disease, and the on-staff psychologist recommended testing for *Streptococcus*, as he suspected that Hannah had developed PANDAS as a result of untreated Strep throat. The throat culture was positive for Strep, which was effectively treated with antibiotics. Further testing by her primary care doctor revealed additional infections at play, including high IgM *Herpes simplex* titers and positive findings for yeast. Upon presenting to our office, Hannah's treatment plan had included a short course of steroids, Augmentin, and Azithromycin.

Signs and Symptoms

In addition to the symptoms her parents had reported during our initial conversation, a more detailed history found that Hannah was also experiencing headaches and itchiness all over her body.

Analysis

After meeting Hannah and hearing her story, I fully agreed with her medical team's initial findings. Still, I felt certain there were other aspects to her Basal Ganglia Encephalitis presentation that needed to be addressed. Additional testing showed positive folate-binding antibody (FRAT), elevated yeast and mold markers, continued positive Strep titers, low vitamin D, and mold exposure with positive urine mycotoxin, very high levels of ochratoxin, and gliotoxin.

Treatment Plan

Adding to the regimen prescribed by her pediatrician, I prescribed Cholestyramine for her elevated ochratoxin, an herbal formula to address the mold and mycotoxin exposure, and vitamin D and foundational immune support. On her first visit, I immediately began glutathione and n-acetyl cysteine treatment for gliotoxin[489]. Her family also thoroughly remediated their home.

Progress Report

Hannah's parents reported that very soon after the new treatment protocol was implemented, she found relief from the headaches and constant itching and that the frequency and intensity of her behavioral flares had significantly decreased. She and her parents were very pleased with how well she was doing—and then a global pandemic hit. Her family relocated to another area less affected by COVID-19, and although she continued to maintain her progress for a time, her headaches and behavioral changes reemerged.

While there is certainly some degree of normalcy to the flare of children's symptoms in times of major stress (and a global pandemic is a major stressor!), I wanted to investigate if this was caused by a new infection, lack of glutathione, or other essential nutrients, or new mold exposure in their new home. I prescribed additional rounds of glutathione and N-acetyl cysteine (a glutathione precursor) for aggressive antioxidant support, which immediately relieved her symptoms. Mold found in their second home was immediately remediated, and Hannah continues to improve.

PANDAS, Mold, Babesia, and Dysautonomia: Zevin

Initial Presentation

- Sudden onset of anxiety, motor tics

- Progression into vocal tics, OCD, and rage

- Worsening and changing of symptoms despite aggressive treatment

Past Medical History

- Healthy pregnancy, delivery, infancy, and early childhood

Dr. O'Hara's Notes

Zevin initially came to us as a three-year-old boy who had developed a compulsion to hop instead of walking following antibiotic treatment for Strep. He suddenly became anxious, particularly about thunder, and his mother, a psychologist, was concerned about PANDAS. After an initial workup, her suspicions about PANDAS were confirmed, and Zevin was treated successfully with therapy, antibiotics, and immunotherapy. He continued to do well over the next few years with prophylactic antibiotics and nutraceuticals. Flares were manageable, and the family adjusted to their new normal.

Fast forward to nine-year-old Zevin. He suddenly developed vocal tics, extreme OCD, and rages. His academic life began to suffer, as he could no longer write his own name or perform basic addition or subtraction, despite being in an advanced math class in previous weeks. He began making noises and constantly rearranging his desk, so it aligned "just right" with the floor tiles. Watching television and reading at home became a stressor because he would have to watch and repeat everything in his head. He reported to me that his "family was a mess and PANDAS was awful."

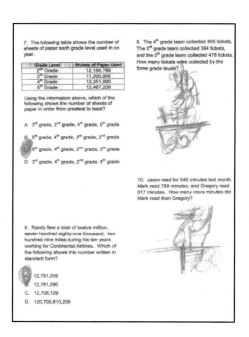

Abrupt Onset of Handwriting OCD

Despite prophylactic antibiotic use and no evidence of sore throat or fever, Zevin was clearly experiencing a significant flare of his Basal Ganglia Encephalitis and, at this time, was found to have evidence of a red anal ring on exam and culture-positive perianal Strep. We changed his antibiotics to Cefdinir and then decided to trial a month-long burst of steroids with great success. Zevin reported that he felt the best he had in years and that his teachers were dumbstruck with his sudden ability to calculate advanced math problems again.

Unfortunately, once the steroids were discontinued, Zevin's PANDAS symptoms returned. Because he had responded so well to steroids, immunoglobulin therapy was recommended. Zevin subsequently had his tonsils and adenoids removed and underwent IVIG. He responded well to IVIG performed every six weeks, reporting minimal OCD, resolution of anxiety, improved social skills, stable mood, and no brain fog.

As Zevin entered high school, however, he began to experience emotional dysregulation and head pain, and his OCD became crippling. Slowly, he also developed dysautonomia—dysregulation of the autonomic nervous system—which appeared as the inability to regulate body temperature, constant dizziness and lightheadedness, and significant night sweats. He was already on nutraceuticals, antiviral and antimicrobial herbs, anti-inflammatories, and IVIG, so this regression was concerning, more subacute than most recognized PANDAS flares. However, one of the culprits revealed itself soon enough, as Zevin's mother found black dots along the AC vent in his room, corroborating our concern about mold and CIRS (see CIRS chapter for further information).

Treatment for this included mold remediation of the family's home and a full purge of paper products in the house, as porous substances are hidden harborers of mold. Medically, we ran tests to determine the exact strain of mold mycotoxin (aspergillus and ochratoxin, in this case) affecting Zevin and the medication recommended to treat it (Cholestyramine). We also found a second culprit of his recent regression, as he tested positive for Babesia, a Lyme co-infection, which is often associated with severe night sweats and air hunger, as well as other symptoms as presented in the chapter on Lyme and Lyme co-infections.

Zevin describes his experience during this time:

"I couldn't talk to friends. I had pain everywhere, and my OCD symptoms never stopped. I couldn't make sense of anything, let alone explain it to others. My guidance counselor was one of the few people in school who understood it, although he thought I was high one day when I walked in to see him because my pupils were so dilated from my symptoms. After school, it took me hours and hours to get through my work, and my showers took me an hour and a half on average. I was freezing when I showered and had to wash myself in a certain way. There wasn't enough time in the day between my work, all my symptoms, and my long showers to get everything done before one in the morning."

During treatment, Zevin was traveling and fell ill with a fever, which was the first time he had experienced an acute illness in five years. This triggered the worst bout of symptoms he had ever experienced, including frank psychosis. This flare was triggered by a viral infection and resolved quickly with a steroid burst and other appropriate interventions.

Analysis

When initially evaluating a childlike 3-year-old Zevin, we begin as indicated in the PANS/PANDAS Functional Medicine Treatment Flowchart, starting with antibiotics or herbal antimicrobials for the identified germ (in his case, Strep), natural immunotherapy (such as anti-inflammatory support, Ibuprofen, hemp oil, quercetin, EFAs, and others), and therapy or other supplemental support of major symptoms. Then, if a child is not improving or there are other significant flares, we consider more invasive interventions, such as steroid bursts followed by HDCs (helminth therapy) if appropriate, IVIG, or plasmapheresis, and finally, if warranted by exam and history, tonsillectomy and/or adenoidectomy.

Often, when a child responds positively to steroids, this indicates that they may respond well to IVIG if needed. If a child has recurrent Strep throat, obstructive sleep apnea, or significant findings on ENT exam, a tonsillectomy and adenoidectomy is pursued. At each crossroad, I return to the questions that Dr. Baker taught me, "Have we done enough for this child?" and "What am I missing?" In Zevin's case, we kept exploring, following his symptoms, and corroborating with laboratory tests to uncover multiple triggers and appropriate treatments. Zevin's is a complicated case, requiring multiple practitioners in his care plan. He had multiple antecedents and many layers to unfold, assess, and treat, and as Zevin often said: "We just keep swimming."

Treatment Plan

With all of his diagnoses, including PANDAS, CIRS from mold/mycotoxin disease, Lyme co-infections (Babesia), and postural orthostatic tachycardia syndrome (POTS) and dysautonomia, we incorporated a comprehensive treatment plan of therapeutic and prophylactic antibiotics, herbal antimicrobials (including those covering viruses and Babesia), probiotics and Saccharomyces, detoxification, supportive nutraceuticals, cannabidiols for his OCD, Cholestyramine, and a beta-blocker for the dysautonomia.

Progress Report

Because of this extensive support, including Cognitive Behavioral Therapy and psychiatric interventions, Zevin began responding. He still struggles significantly with symptoms, including head pain, dysautonomia symptoms, OCD, and perseverative thoughts. Still, he has been able to play classical jazz piano competitively and was admitted to his first-choice college. Together with his care team, we continue to look for answers and interventions for Zevin.

Summary

Zevin's case is complicated, but because I specialize in caring for children with Basal Ganglia Encephalitis and often complex presentations, Zevin is not alone in our practice. This disease is about the lack of immune tolerance. Our children with more complex or prolonged presentations may have multiple triggers, germs, and immunologic, metabolic, neuropsychiatric, and other derailments. Like Zevin, they may require multiple interventions, an experienced care team, and ongoing support for the entire family during the severe episodic course of this disease.

OCD/POTS:
KRISTEN

Initial Presentation

- Headaches

- Lightheadedness

- Nausea

- Palpitations

- Fatigue

- Discoloration of lower extremities

Past Medical History

- Healthy and normal infancy and early childhood

- OCD surrounding thoughts of accidents began at age 10

- Thrush

- Vaginal yeast infections

- History of mild Raynaud's syndrome

Kristen had a previous medical history of thrush and diaper rashes in infancy and, later, vaginal yeast infections in childhood. Other than these, previous medical history and exams were all normal.

After multiple failed SSRIs, her OCD was originally controlled by a previous physician with n-acetyl cysteine (NAC), an excellent intervention for OCD. Studies show that NAC helps with compulsive gambling, nail-biting, skin picking, etc., and we're also seeing improvements in irritability and anxiety for those with Autism Spectrum Disorder. (see the earlier chapter on OCD). Kristen's previous doctor also encouraged mindfulness exercises to help with the OCD and treated her tendency toward yeast infections with a rotation of various herbs, broad-spectrum probiotics, and the more targeted yeast-like strain of *Saccharomyces boulardii*, with success.

Family Medical History

- Mother has celiac disease, episcleritis, and Raynaud's syndrome
- Paternal grandparents have arthritis, colitis, and asthma

Dr. O'Hara's Notes

Kristen came to me as a fourteen-year-old with chronic headaches. She was a pleasant young woman who came into the office with both of her parents. She had a fairly normal history and healthy childhood. She is a twin, born by cesarean section, had normal development in her early years, and was raised by a very functional and loving family. She first presented to another physician with severe OCD at age ten. She would repeat things over and over, and she had repeated thoughts of accidents that she could not ignore. She developed rituals around these thoughts of accidents every time she left the house and had extreme anxiety until her rituals could be completed. She would check on everyone continually.

Signs and Symptoms

Taking a more detailed history brought to light Kristen's complaints of lightheadedness, nausea, palpitations, abdominal pain, fatigue, and rashes, in addition to the chief complaint of headaches that she had initially reported. Physical exam showed significant blood pressure and heart rate changes as outlined below, as well as significant Raynaud's and lower extremity discoloration.

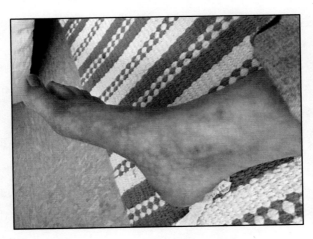

Marked Lower Extremity Discoloration

Laboratory Tests

When she finally came to see me, all initial labs were normal (thyroid, ANA, infectious disease, blood counts, etc.). The only findings of note were low levels of zinc and magnesium.

Analysis

In Kristen's case, it was important for me to categorize her symptoms by diagnoses she already had, those I was considering, and those that did not necessarily fit either of them. The following is a breakdown of my thought process.

- Symptoms consistent with yeast overgrowth: none currently (well treated)

- Additional symptoms: dizziness, fatigue, heart palpitations, nausea, headaches

- Differential diagnoses: dysautonomia or POTS (dysregulation of any of the autonomic or somatic nervous system processes), adrenal insufficiency, hormonal/pubertal changes given her age, atypical migraines (can present with neurologic changes, nausea, and abdominal pain), cardiovascular disease (ruled out by extensive physical exam and cardiology review)

Kristen's history was consistent with dysautonomia, which can be easily confirmed in-office with basic physical tests. I performed Valsalva maneuvers (blowing against resistance) and further tested her autonomic nervous system with blood pressures taken standing and sitting. She had definitive results with blood pressures of 110/70 mm Hg when sitting and 90/60 mm Hg upon standing. During all of these tests, she noted that she felt an increase in nausea and a "racing heart." She was diagnosed with and confirmed to have postural orthostatic tachycardia syndrome (POTS).[490]

Treatment Plan

To manage her POTS/dysautonomia,[491] her treatment plan included:

- Vitamin B12 to support the normal production of adrenaline and improve adrenal function, specifically to combat her fatigue, brain fog, and nausea.[492]

- Increased filtered water intake to at least 1 oz/kg per day

- Increased salt consumption (I prefer iodized sea salt or Himalayan pink salt)

- Lifestyle modifications to prevent syncope and dizziness, including:

  o Avoiding standing or sitting for extended periods of time

  o Wearing compression tights and/or an abdominal binder

  o Moderate exercise focused on isotonic exercises

  o Adequate sleep focused on improved sleep hygiene, including:

    - Dark room, no blue light, weighted blanket, cold temperature.

    - Supplementation with melatonin to further support normal and healthy sleep, with the additional benefits of antioxidant support.

Working closely with a nutritionist, Kristen also avoided all processed food (specifically those high in nitrates and preserved with BHA or BHT—think pepperoni, salami, etc.), hydrogenated fats, commercial stocks/broths/soups/seasonings, MSG, canned and dried foods, and artificial sweeteners. She was encouraged to eat as organically as possible, focusing on the "Clean 15" and avoiding the "Dirty Dozen" (though now at least the "Dirty Fifteen"), as recommended by the Environmental Working Group.

Although these weren't necessary in Kristen's case, pharmaceuticals can be considered for many of the symptoms of POTS, including management with Fludrocortisone, Scopolamine, Midodrine, or beta-blockers; stimulants for brain fog and fatigue; Mestinon for early satiety and nausea; Remeron or Clonidine for sleep; and antimicrobials for dysbiosis (typically SIBO or yeast overgrowth).

Progress Report

After three months on this treatment plan, Kristen's dizziness and syncope improved, but she still complained of mild nausea, occasional heart palpitations, and headaches with extended exertion. We added *Glycyrrhiza glabra*, licorice root, to further decrease inflammation and soothe her GI tract, which alleviated the remaining nausea. (Note: licorice root can increase blood pressure and deplete potassium, so monitor these closely.) We also added magnesium glycinate to help stabilize her vasculature and minimize headaches. Complementary therapies such as osteopathic manipulation, craniosacral therapy, and chiropractic medicine were extremely helpful in managing Kristen's remaining POTS symptoms.

As of the time of this writing, Kristin maintains an ongoing foundational care plan of diet and lifestyle changes, paying close attention to salt and hydration, maintenance doses of vitamin B12, NAC for her OCD, probiotics, including *Saccharomyces boulardii* for yeast, magnesium, CoQ10, and melatonin. She continues to do well and is just completing college.

Tics and Antioxidants: Caleb

Initial Presentation

- Verbal and motor tics

- Anxiety

- Aggression

- Frequent urination

Past Medical History

- Possible mild rash and reaction to MMR vaccination

- Reported sore throat

- Otherwise previously healthy

Caleb's past history included a healthy and normal pregnancy and birth. He was breastfed, initially with poor latching. He was healthy, with few infections and normal developmental milestones. Caleb had some sensory processing issues, as he was somewhat more sensitive to noises and sometimes had trouble modulating his moods. Still, he never received a diagnosis or treatment for these previously. He ate an organic diet, had no known pesticide or toxic exposures, no past surgeries or major injuries, had never received anesthesia, and no previous lab tests had been performed until his pediatrician began investigating PANDAS.

Family Medical History

- Positive Strep culture in sibling around the same time his behavioral changes began

Caleb's extended family medical history included arthritis, insulin-dependent diabetes, and cancer.

Dr. O'Hara's Notes

Caleb is a healthy 5-year-old with a new onset of tics. He had a sudden onset of vocal tics, saying "excuse me" every five seconds at variable pitches, tones, and volumes, including during sleep initiation. He also developed motor tics, which involved scratching and smelling his buttocks and touching his shoulder in a repetitive sequence. His family saw a dramatic change in his personality, as he became much more anxious and aggressive toward his sister and began putting everything in his mouth. He had an abrupt onset of all of these symptoms and was very distressed by them.

Upon presenting to our office, Caleb had recently received his first MMR vaccine. About one and a half weeks later, he developed violent vomiting, rash, and fever for two days but had no other symptoms related to vaccination. He had no known Lyme tick exposures and no other infectious disease exposures or symptoms. His sister had culture-positive Strep throat, but his culture was negative. His pediatrician thought it might be PANS or PANDAS, so they placed him on a course of Azithromycin, but this resulted in no change in his tics. He then trialed Amoxicillin-Clavulanate, again with no improvement. The pediatrician also performed some initial blood work, including ASO and antiDNase B antibody, a Lyme screen and western blot, CBC, and sed rate, all of which were normal at that time.

Signs and Symptoms

His exam was entirely normal except for the almost constant tics.

Analysis

As Caleb and his family presented to our office, I mulled over the laundry list of causes of neuropsychiatric inflammation—PANDAS, PANS, Lyme or a coinfection, viruses, other bacterial infections, and other potential medical or metabolic complications that could be at play, including seizures, new onset of Tourette's, metabolic issues, abuse, trauma, medication or drug overdose, and late-onset of autism. Because all of these were possibilities, we decided to run a comprehensive set of labs to investigate them, including a repeat of the bloodwork that his pediatrician had ordered, as sometimes blood titers are negative if tested too early in the progression of the disease. We included better testing of his Lyme, Strep, Mycoplasma, and appropriate viral titers, CBC, CMP, liver, and kidney function markers, mitochondrial markers because of the poor initial latching, CRP and ANA as inflammatory markers, vitamin A, vitamin D, MMA as a measure of B12, and a cysteine level as a measure of glutathione status. He had a recent MRI and EEG, ordered by his pediatrician, as well as drug testing, all of which were normal.

Test Results

All of that testing came back entirely normal (including a negative Strep culture), except for his cysteine level, which was very low. Normal on this particular lab should be greater than one, and his level was measured at 0.36.

Initial Treatment Plan

Because Caleb had been on an antibiotic previously, we immediately started him on a restorative probiotic and recommended essential fatty acids as an initial anti-inflammatory intervention. We also decided to administer glutathione. Although this is not protocol for many of our patients, we will sometimes immediately give glutathione because it has been reported in the literature that there is an association between glutathione and tardive dyskinesia[493] and that it may quickly resolve involuntary movements.[494] In our anecdotal experience, we have seen improvements with oral n-acetyl cysteine, a precursor of glutathione, as well as glutathione, in effectively managing tics, anxiety, and OCD.

Progress Report

Caleb returned two weeks later, and his mother reported that his tics completely resolved after the first round of glutathione. His behavior had normalized, he had no further anxiety, he was not experiencing bouts of aggression, and he had stopped hurting his sister and himself.

Because all of his labs were normal except for the cysteine, we decided to place him on continued methylation support. His treatment plan focused on broccoli seed extract as a potent source of the antioxidant compound sulforaphane, n-acetyl cysteine, glycine, an additional precursor of glutathione, and methylated B vitamins, including MeTHF. We continued the probiotics and essential fatty acids and focused on supporting his antioxidant capacity.

Summary

This child has lived an extremely "clean" life with many protective factors, including healthy and normal pregnancy and birth, exclusive breastfeeding, and a generally organic lifestyle. We postulate that he had a genetic susceptibility to low glutathione levels and unfortunately fielded multiple triggers within a short period of time: mild reaction to the MMR vaccine, sore throat potentially caused by another viral infection, and exposure to his sibling's Strep throat. In our opinion, the intense combination of these depleted his glutathione levels and created stress and inflammation in his nervous system, triggering tics, anxiety, and aggression. In building up his glutathione stores, we were able to help him to resolve the neurobehavioral symptoms by improving his body's ability to detoxify.

After explaining our approach to his family, Caleb continued natural glutathione support for some time until his family felt comfortable in weaning him from this protocol. His family now turns to n-acetyl cysteine and other methylation interventions whenever he has a virus, encounters any other triggers, or develops any mild neurobehavioral symptoms, with much success. Currently, his supplementation regimen includes probiotics, essential fatty acids, and a B vitamin complex—a manageable and appropriate long-term combination for this child, in our opinion.

PANDAS, Crohn's, and HDCs: Charlie

Initial Presentation

- Anxiety
- GI complaints

Past Medical History

- Diagnosed with Autism Spectrum Disorder at age three
- Recent history of Strep infection

Family Medical History

His mother and several other family members have anxiety.

Dr. O'Hara's Notes

Charlie was diagnosed with Autism Spectrum Disorder at the age of three. He had remarkable improvements at that time with a gluten-free, casein-free, soy-free, and sugar-free diet and had further improvements with speech, occupational, and behavioral therapy. He was not on any prescription medications, but basic biomedical interventions had helped with symptom management.

When Charlie presented to my office at age nine, he had a sudden onset of increased anxiety. He had recently recovered from a Strep infection, and his mother was seeking answers to his changed behavior. He was also experiencing loose stools and mild abdominal cramping, especially after eating.

Signs and Symptoms

Physical examination, including an abdominal exam, was within normal limits.

Laboratory Tests

The following tests were positive:

- Occult blood in stool

- High ASO (780) and antiDNaseB Ab (910)

- Positive ANA (antinuclear antibodies) at 1:320.

No other elevations or abnormalities were found at that time.

Analysis

Because of his GI complaints and occult blood in his stool, Charlie was referred to a gastroenterologist to rule out GI pathology, who cleared him of any GI issues. However, the abrupt onset of his anxiety, high Strep titers, and positive ANA led us to consider a trial of antimicrobials to treat him for possible PANDAS and determine if there was a resolution or improvement in his anxiety.

Treatment Plan

To minimize GI irritation and because it is known to potentially resolve symptoms quickly, we decided to prescribe intramuscular Bicillin rather than oral antibiotics. With this treatment, his anxiety immediately improved.

Progress Report

Charlie did well with this initial round of treatment for the Strep infection. In fact, four years passed until he presented to our office again at age 13. Just as before, increasing anxiety was his leading symptom. His mother had been treating him with hemp oil but noted that he had a fifteen-pound weight loss, loose stools, and a marked decrease in appetite.

When he returned to our office at that time, we found that Charlie had a slightly distended belly with mild diffuse tenderness. We ran blood work and a stool analysis, which was positive for occult blood, elevated lysozyme, and high fecal calprotectin, indicating inflammation. Blood work showed that his C-reactive protein was 46; our local lab's normal reference range for this marker is less than 1.

We immediately referred Charlie to a gastroenterologist and started him on a GI-healing protocol, which included probiotics, *Saccharomyces boulardii*, and an herbal rotation including oil of oregano and caprylic acid, and grapefruit seed extract. He continued on the hemp oil, and we added 5-HTP for agitation and anxiety.

The gastroenterologist performed a colonoscopy, and he was diagnosed, as expected, with Crohn's disease. Because of the weight loss, decreased appetite, and loose stools, his medical team and family decided to treat Crohn's aggressively. He was initially placed on 5-Aminosalicylic acid and a brief course of Metronidazole. Although his gastroenterologist wanted to put him on Methotrexate, Charlie was not fully vaccinated. It was decided that he needed to complete his vaccinations before beginning any further immunosuppressive medications. His mother was paralyzed with fear and did not want to use Methotrexate due to the possible significant side effects.

The family agreed to begin the vaccination regimen before starting Methotrexate, which was estimated to take three months to complete. Given this delay, we decided to introduce HDCs, in hopes of reconstituting his microbiome and promoting immune tolerance in the meantime. You can read more on the background and uses for HDCs in the HDC chapter. Still, in short, modern industrialized culture (water treatment, toilets, using antibacterial soaps and detergents, lack of outdoor exposure, etc.) has depleted the diversity and vigor of our microbiomes. This increases, in part, the wide range of autoimmune diseases we see in modern times, including Inflammatory Bowel Diseases. After an extensive review of the literature, HDCs were considered for Charlie to help manage the inflammation associated with Crohn's.

When helminths were introduced and increased gradually over the course of several weeks, Charlie had no negative reactions to this treatment, and his chronic pain decreased. Over the course of three months, he gained eighteen pounds, his stools normalized, and his appetite improved, as did his anxiety. Charlie's family was very hesitant to discuss the HDCs treatment with his gastroenterologist, who, not knowing that the HDCs had been started, did not have a good explanation on why Charlie was making such good progress but was happy, nonetheless. After three years of monitoring, Charlie continued to gain weight normally, had normalized stools, and all labs returned to persistently normal limits.

Although the medical team involved in his care created a comprehensive treatment plan for Charlie, I believe that his abrupt return to health was in large part due to HDCs. This intervention is an indicated and research-proven treatment for gastrointestinal diseases but is also successful in managing neuropsychological issues resulting from autoimmune disease. Please refer to our mentoring program as well as the earlier chapter on HDCs Therapy for references and further information.

Autism and HDCs:
Ty

Initial Presentation

- Rage

- Anxiety with skin picking

- Enuresis

- Handwriting deterioration

Past Medical History

- Autism Spectrum Disorder, diagnosed at age 2

Dr. O'Hara's Notes

Ty is a 13-year-old boy with autism. He is minimally verbal, with repetitive OCD behaviors, minor sleep disruption, and difficulty with social interaction. When he was twelve years old, he developed abrupt onset behavioral changes with severe outbursts of rage, skin picking, overwhelming anxiety, handwriting deterioration, sleep disruption, and severe enuresis. He had previously been potty trained and did not have a history of bedwetting but suddenly developed both nighttime and daytime enuresis.

Physical Exam

Physical examination was within normal limits.

Laboratory Tests

Throat and rectal cultures for Strep were performed, which were negative. Liver, kidney, and thyroid function and antibodies were all normal, as were Strep titers, Lyme western blot, and co-infections. However, Ty had a minimally elevated ANA, 1:160, in a diffuse pattern with a negative reflex panel. Although he had not been sick with pneumonia or sinusitis, his Mycoplasma titers were very high, with a positive IFA, an IgM of 2150, and an IgG of 3.5.

Analysis

The differential diagnosis included normal pubertal changes, seizures, Lyme, mold, metabolic issues like thyroid or adrenal dysfunction, medication or drug overdose, trauma, abuse, and of course, neuroinflammation of PANS and PANDAS. Because of the marked evidence of Mycoplasma infection and inflammation, and most importantly, because of the abrupt onset of enuresis coupled with rage and anxiety, we diagnosed him with PANS and moved forward with antibiotic treatment after eliminating other pertinent diagnoses.

Treatment

Azithromycin immediately improved Ty's symptoms, with only occasional skin picking remaining. Ty's symptoms of autism were unchanged by this treatment. Still, because of his improvement with the neurobehavioral issues and enuresis, we decided to maintain him on weekly Azithromycin, commonly used as a prophylactic treatment. We ordered an EKG to ensure he did not have a prolonged QT interval, which was normal.

Progress Report

After several months without consultation, his parents discontinued the prophylactic Azithromycin, and he developed a sinus infection. This sparked an increase in OCD, specifically, biting himself until his skin bled. Both his bloodwork and his family's cultures were negative at that time. Repeated courses of antibiotics, including Amoxicillin, Amoxicillin-Clavulanate, Clindamycin, and Ciprofloxacin, were trialed by his pediatrician with no change. Ty would not tolerate any herbs and refused all other nutraceuticals at that time.

We had many questions about his current situation. Was this still PANS? What else could we still be missing? His Strep and Mycoplasma titers and urine organic acid at this time were normal. His ANA, however, was elevated, as it was now 1:320 in a diffuse pattern. We decided to do advanced testing through Moleculera's Cunningham Panel and found that his Cam Kinase level was markedly elevated at 206. Though we only utilize this test in atypical or hard-to-diagnose cases, this was a prime example of how this test can help with management in cases like Ty's. His elevation was consistent with Strep-induced Basal Ganglia Encephalitis (or PANDAS) and helped us to continue to find appropriate treatments for him.

We gave him one dose of intramuscular LA-Bicillin, and his family reported marked improvement. Unfortunately, he and his parents subsequently declined further intramuscular Bicillin because it was very painful, so we needed to find another option. Although he had inflammation, he was not getting better with the usual antibiotics and immune modulation, and IVIG was not an option because of cost and lack of insurance approval. He did not improve with steroids.

Multiple SSRIs and antipsychotics were trialed, but his condition worsened on these: his OCD became extreme, he was not sleeping because of his anxiety, and he was literally climbing the walls. Rather than focus on "killing the pathogen" or trialing more SSRI or antipsychotic medications, we decided to focus on immunotherapies, including curcumin, quercetin, and resveratrol, among others. We also decided to try helminth therapy/HDCs. Immediately after introducing the HDCs, he was calmer, slept through the night without enuresis, began to eat well, had no agitation or anxiety, and was much more interactive with adults and other children.

HDCs Balance the Biome

Although you can read more about HDCs in the chapter dedicated to them, I will briefly summarize their mechanism of action. HDCs are grain beetle worm eggs that have been shown to promote immune tolerance through the stimulation of Th2, essentially retraining the immune system to be less reactive. This reconstitution of our biome may help to decrease inflammatory disorders and promote immune tolerance. The benefits of HDCs are that they are low cost, there is no risk of transmission from human to human, the distribution of HDCs is strictly intraluminal (inside the gut), and they do not breach the barrier of the gut like hookworms and whipworms can.

HDC Clinical Concerns

Of note, there may be an inflammatory response similar to a Herxheimer reaction or healing crisis when we begin HDCs. If this occurs, administration of an antihistamine and an anti-inflammatory like Ibuprofen can help control this reaction. Slow titration with an experienced practitioner is necessary to prevent further aggravations.

There is a very slight chance of infestation (not infection) if the HDCs (the eggs) hatch, so we do not want to use this intervention in children with constipation or slow GI transit time, who take immunocompromising medications, or who already have symptoms of severe cramping or abdominal pain. We may also want to avoid HDCs in nonverbal patients, as they cannot communicate if they have severe cramping or pain. The chance of infestation is 0.1% but increased in children with immunosuppression or constipation. If an infestation occurs, it is treated very quickly with Biltricide at 20 mg per kg per day, in three divided doses over the course of one day.

Finally, HDCs are unlike bacteria: they do not multiply inside the body. They also cannot adapt like bacteria, so they will always be sensitive to Biltricide.

In general, if you have a child with OCD, anxiety, severe allergic or autoimmune disease, you will want to first treat constipation, remove any stressors (food, allergens, toxins), and supply appropriate nutrients that they may need. Introduction of anti-inflammatories such as Ibuprofen, flavonoids, essential fatty acids, prescription steroids, curcumin, or quercetin to decrease the neuroinflammation should also be considered. Treat any underlying germ overgrowth with antimicrobials, and look for any underlying conditions that may be contributing to the disease process, including other causes of the behavioral and neuropsychiatric symptoms.

Summary

I believe HDCs helped diminish Ty's most severe symptoms, eliminated his rage and enuresis, decreased his anxiety and OCD, and helped him function in his day-to-day life. Ty is still autistic, but more importantly, he is happier, healthier, and calmer without multiple medications or expensive interventions.

PANS AND COVID: LAYLA

Initial Presentation

- Emotional volatility
- Intrusive and looping thoughts
- Jerking movements in the pelvis and lower spine

Past Medical History

Six weeks prior to the onset of the symptoms, Layla was exposed to COVID at school. As a result, she and her sister experienced transient diarrhea, as well as loss of taste and smell. Other than these mild symptoms, her course of COVID infection was uncomplicated and resolved within several days. After several weeks though, mom noted that her toes had become red and swollen.

Family Medical History

Layla's sister was diagnosed with *Mycoplasma pneumoniae* three years prior to her presentation to my office. Mom had been previously treated for Babesia prior to pregnancy with Layla but reported no known negative effects on gestation because of it and no residual symptoms in herself.

Dr. O'Hara's Notes

Ten-year-old Layla was always a spunky, lively, and athletic girl with a proclivity for organization and order. However, on February 15, 2021, her behavior and personality "became something else entirely," according to her parents. She went from being an emotionally balanced child to one with constant intrusive thoughts looping all day long. She became emotionally volatile and presented to our office crying, begging for us to help her, saying she would rather die than go through another day of this. She began experiencing jerking movements in her pelvis or lower spine. The movements occurred all day, and she even experienced them while falling asleep some nights. These symptoms would wane and then become extreme from one day to the next. Both Doxycycline and Fluoxetine were started before I began seeing Layla for concerns about Lyme and depression, but she saw minimal resolution or improvement in her symptoms with these medications.

Physical Exam and Testing

At the time of our visit, six weeks after her symptoms first began, Layla continued to experience emotional lability and pelvic twitching. Physical examination demonstrated the classic "COVID toes" of MISC-C but was otherwise within normal limits. Laboratory evidence was positive for inflammation, with a mildly positive ANA and ESR, and was positive for COVID IgG antibodies. She also had evidence of low vitamin A, vitamin D, and RBC zinc. Strep, Mycoplasma, Lyme, and Lyme co-infection panels were all negative, as was further work-up.

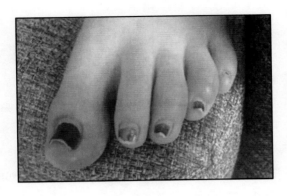

COVID toes (MISC-C With Swelling and Erythema of Distal Toes)

Analysis

Viruses are among the most common triggers of PANS. Although neurobehavioral changes were not reported as a common symptom of COVID-19 infection at the time of Layla's presentation, we knew that this virus caused widespread inflammation. In this case, COVID may have triggered neuroinflammation in Layla's brain and, therefore, her neurobehavioral symptoms. We decided to provide comprehensive immune support and general antiviral therapy to see if it would resolve Layla's symptoms and explore further diagnostics if this treatment had no effect.

Treatment

Essential fatty acids (EFAs), curcumin (a potent anti-inflammatory), and resveratrol (an antioxidant) were introduced to calm her neuroinflammation. We also recommended lysine and monolaurin as natural antivirals. Given the insufficiencies found in her blood work, we added antioxidants, including vitamins A, D, and zinc, which further supported her healthy immune function.

Follow-Up

At follow-up six weeks later, her overall mood was less volatile. She had more stamina and a more positive outlook and reported feeling much more like herself. Given the positive COVID antibodies and the timeline, we are postulating that COVID-19 was the triggering factor for her abrupt onset of symptoms. Diarrhea, smell, and taste changes can be the only presenting factors for children. We continue to monitor Layla, providing ongoing therapeutic support, as well as discussing antiviral and immunologic support for any future viral infections. Because we know it causes MIS-C and post-COVID inflammation in a limited subset of children, COVID-19 may be another triggering factor for PANS, and we need to consider heavily moving forward.

Additional Thoughts on COVID-Related PANS

Now that we are farther into the COVID pandemic than when Layla first presented, a large amount of research is illuminating some of the neurobehavioral effects COVID has had on children and adults, such as cerebral ischaemic stroke, intracerebral hemorrhages, encephalopathy, and cerebral vasculitis.[495] Ageusia, anosmia, myalgia, paraesthesia, and Guillain-Barré syndrome are the most reported disorders affecting the peripheral nervous system in patients with COVID-19.[496]

Pavone et al. documented two unrelated adolescents with a clinical diagnosis of new-onset PANS who had been diagnosed with COVID-19 via nasal swab two weeks before symptom onset. The children experienced the abrupt onset of neurobehavioral symptoms similar to those seen in children with Mycoplasma or other viral-induced cases of PANS.[497]

The mechanism of COVID-19's impact on neurological impairment is not precisely known, but a few colleagues have presented some hypotheses. First, they hypothesized a direct viral injury to neural cells through olfactory nerves and its transit to the CNS via the cribriform plate. The second hypothesis is that SARS-CoV-2 causes vascular endothelial injury through its interaction with angiotensin-converting enzyme 2 receptors. Finally, they have hypothesized that COVID-19 causes inflammatory and autoimmune injury. COVID-19, in its most serious manifestations, presents with aberrant and excessive inflammation mediated by innate and adaptive immune activation.[498]

Although not a common cause of PANS, it would be a mistake to exclude COVID-19 from a list of differentials when considering viral-induced illness. In light of a global pandemic with ever-evolving variants, we must be aware of the potential neuroinflammatory impact this virus may have on our children.

EPILOGUE

In researching and writing this book with my editor, Sarah Ouano, ND, I gained even more understanding and appreciation of this complex and devastating disease. I hope this book has helped you better understand and broaden your perspective of PANS, PANDAS, and Basal Ganglia Encephalitis. I hope you will remember the three-pronged approach of treating the underlying infectious or metabolic triggers, utilizing immunomodulation and immune support, and assessing and treating the symptoms, starting with those of greatest impact on the child and family. After a thorough history, physical exam, and appropriate laboratory testing, as an allopathic physician faced with a child with abrupt onset of neuropsychiatric symptoms, I will start with treating the infectious triggers with antibiotics such as Azithromycin, Cefdinir, Penicillin, and sometimes Amoxicillin-Clavulanate, Tetracyclines, or others. As a functional medicine practitioner, I will consider all antimicrobials and all forms of immunomodulation, in addition to Ibuprofen, steroids, and immunomodulating medications. As a clinician, I use all research at my disposal to inform the care of each child and family. As a healer, I will use all the tools in my toolbox to treat all facets of this disease and, most importantly, to allay the devastating symptoms of OCD, tics, anxiety, rage, cognitive, sleep, and urinary issues. As a detective, I will keep digging, searching, and trying to find the answers for each child using all modalities available to me, my colleagues, and this child and family. As a mom and a teacher, I will listen and support and learn and never quit.

I hope this book inspires you to work with these families. It can be a challenging but exceedingly rewarding endeavor. If you are interested, reach out to me. If you want to learn more about nutraceuticals, herbals, their dosing, usages, and other integrative therapies, check out our programs. We would be happy to help you move forward on this healing journey for you, your families, and your practice.

In health,

Nancy

www.drohara.com

DISCLAIMER

The content of this guidebook is provided for informational purposes only. It is in no way intended as medical advice, a substitute for medical counseling, or as treatment or cure for any disease or health condition. Always work with a qualified health professional before making any changes to your diet, supplement use, prescription drug use, lifestyle, or exercise activities. Readers assume all risks from the use, non-use, or misuse of the information herein.

ABOUT THE AUTHOR

Dr. Nancy O'Hara is a board-certified Pediatrician. Her career is dedicated to caring for children with neurodevelopmental and neuropsychiatric issues. She received her medical degree from The University of Pennsylvania as a member of the Alpha Omega Alpha Honor Society and a Masters in Public Health from the University of Pittsburgh. She

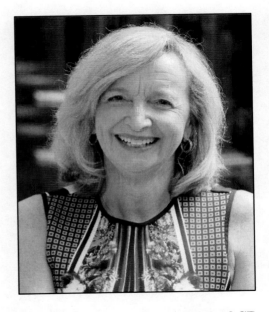

lectures nationally and internationally on PANS/PANDAS/BGE, OCD, Lyme, ASD, and ADHD. Beyond being a clinician and teacher, Dr. O'Hara is blessed to be a mom. She lives in Connecticut with her husband.

INDEX

B

C

F

H

M

O

S

U

V

X

Y

Z

REFERENCES

The PANS/PANDAS Journey

Considering PANDAS

1 Tang, A. W., Appel, H. J., Bennett, S. C., Forsyth, L. H., Glasser, S. K., Jarka, M. A., Kory, P. D., Malik, A. N., Martonoffy, A. I., Wahlin, L. K., Williams, T. T., Woodin, N. A., Woodin, L. C., Miller, I. K. T., & Miller, L. G. (2021). Treatment barriers in PANS/PANDAS: Observations from eleven health care provider families. Families, Systems, & Health, 39(3), 477–487. https://doi.org/10.1037/fsh0000602

2 Wells, Lindsey. (2021). Super Sam and the Battle Against PANS/PANDAS. Self-published.

3 Bodner, S. M., Morshed, S. A., & Peterson, B. S. (2001). The question of PANDAS in Adults. Biological Psychiatry, 49(9), 807–810. https://doi.org/10.1016/s0006-3223(00)01127-6

4 Platt, M. P., Bolding, K. A., Wayne, C. R., Chaudhry, S., Cutforth, T., Franks, K. M., & Agalliu, D. (2020). Th17 lymphocytes drive vascular and neuronal deficits in a mouse model of postinfectious autoimmune encephalitis. Proceedings of the National Academy of Sciences, 117(12), 6708–6716. https://doi.org/10.1073/pnas.1911097117

5 Chain, J. L., Alvarez, K., Mascaro-Blanco, A., Reim, S., Bentley, R., Hommer, R., Grant, P., Leckman, J. F., Kawikova, I., Williams, K., Stoner, J. A., Swedo, S. E., & Cunningham, M. W. (2020). Autoantibody biomarkers for basal ganglia encephalitis in Sydenham chorea and pediatric autoimmune neuropsychiatric disorder associated with Streptococcal infections. Frontiers in Psychiatry, 11, 564. https://doi.org/10.3389/fpsyt.2020.00564

6 Zheng, J, Frankovich J, McKenna ES, et al. (2020). Association of Pediatric Acute-Onset Neuropsychiatric Syndrome With Microstructural Differences in Brain Regions Detected via Diffusion-Weighted Magnetic Resonance Imaging. JAMA Netw Open. 2020; 3(5): e204063. doi:10.1001/jamanetworkopen.2020.4063

7 Baj, J., Sitarz, E., Forma, A., Wróblewska, K., & Karakuła-Juchnowicz, H. (2020). Alterations in the Nervous System and Gut Microbiota after β-Hemolytic Streptococcus Group A Infection-Characteristics and Diagnostic Criteria of PANDAS Recognition. International Journal of Molecular Sciences, 21(4), 1476. https://doi.org/10.3390/ijms21041476

8 Louveau, A., Smirnov, I., Keyes, T. J., Eccles, J. D., Rouhani, S. J., Peske, J. D., Derecki, N. C., Castle, D., Mandell, J. W., Lee, K. S., Harris, T. H., & Kipnis, J. (2015). Structural and functional features of central nervous system lymphatic vessels. Nature, 523(7560), 337–341. https://doi.org/10.1038/nature14432

9 Dileepan, T., Smith, E. D., Knowland, D., Hsu, M., Platt, M., Bittner-Eddy, P., Cohen, B., Southern, P., Latimer, E., Harley, E., Agalliu, D., & Cleary, P. P. (2016). Group A Streptococcus intranasal infection promotes CNS infiltration by Streptococcal-specific Th17 cells. The Journal of Clinical Investigation, 126(1), 303–317. https://doi.org/10.1172/JCI80792

10 Thienemann, M., Murphy, T., Leckman, J., Shaw, R., Williams, K., Kapphahn, C., Frankovich, J., Geller, D., Bernstein, G., Chang, K., Elia, J., & Swedo, S. (2017). Clinical Management of Pediatric Acute-Onset Neuropsychiatric Syndrome: Part I-Psychiatric and Behavioral Interventions. Journal of Child and Adolescent Psychopharmacology, 27(7), 566–573. https://doi.org/10.1089/cap.2016.0145).

11 Swedo, S. E., Seidlitz, J., Kovacevic, M., Latimer, M. E., Hommer, R., Lougee, L., & Grant, P. (2015). Clinical presentation of pediatric autoimmune neuropsychiatric disorders associated with Streptococcal infections in research and community settings. Journal of Child and Adolescent Psychopharmacology, 25(1), 26–30. https://doi.org/10.1089/cap.2014.0073

12 Chang, K., Frankovich, J., Cooperstock, M., Cunningham, M. W., Latimer, M. E., Murphy, T. K., Pasternack, M., Thienemann, M., Williams, K., Walter, J., Swedo, S. E., & PANS Collaborative Consortium. (2015). Clinical evaluation of youth with pediatric acute-onset neuropsychiatric syndrome (PANS): recommendations from the 2013 PANS Consensus Conference. Journal of Child and Adolescent Psychopharmacology, 25(1), 3–13. https://doi.org/10.1089/cap.2014.0084

13 Cox, C. J., Zuccolo, A. J., Edwards, E. V., Mascaro-Blanco, A., Alvarez, K., Stoner, J., Chang, K., & Cunningham, M. W. (2015). Antineuronal antibodies in a heterogeneous group of youth and young adults with tics and obsessive-compulsive disorder. Journal of Child and Adolescent Psychopharmacology, 25(1), 76–85. https://doi.org/10.1089/cap.2014.0048

14 Dalmau, J., Lancaster, E., Martinez-Hernandez, E., Rosenfeld, M. R., & Balice-Gordon, R. (2011). Clinical experience and laboratory investigations in patients with anti-NMDAR encephalitis. The Lancet. Neurology, 10(1), 63–74. https://doi.org/10.1016/S1474-4422(10)70253-2

15 Peng, L., Kang, S., Yin, Z., Jia, R., Song, X., Li, L., Li, Z., Zou, Y., Liang, X., Li, L., He, C., Ye, G., Yin, L., Shi, F., Lv, C., & Jing, B. (2015). Antibacterial activity and mechanism of berberine against Streptococcus agalactiae. International Journal of Clinical and Experimental Pathology, 8(5), 5217–5223.

16 Chava, V. R., Manjunath, S. M., Rajanikanth, A. V., & Sridevi, N. (2012). The efficacy of neem extract on four microorganisms responsible for causing dental caries viz Streptococcus mutans, Streptococcus salivarius, Streptococcus mitis and Streptococcus sanguis: an in vitro study. The Journal of Contemporary Dental Practice, 13(6), 769–772. https://doi.org/10.5005/jp-journals-10024-1227

17 Hobbs, C. (1986). Usnea: The herbal antibiotic and other medicinal lichens. Botanica Press.

18 Srivastava, P., Upreti, D. K., Dhole, T. N., Srivastava, A. K., & Nayak, M. T. (2013). Antimicrobial Property of Extracts of Indian Lichen against Human Pathogenic Bacteria. Interdisciplinary Perspectives on Infectious Diseases, 2013, 709348. https://doi.org/10.1155/2013/709348

19 Dean, S. L., & Singer, H. S. (2017). Treatment of Sydenham's Chorea: A Review of the Current Evidence. Tremor and Other Hyperkinetic Movements (New York, N.Y.), 7, 456. https://doi.org/10.7916/D8W95GJ2

20 Brown, K. D., Farmer, C., Freeman, G. M., Jr, Spartz, E. J., Farhadian, B., Thienemann, M., & Frankovich, J. (2017). Effect of Early and Prophylactic Nonsteroidal Anti-Inflammatory Drugs on Flare Duration in Pediatric Acute-Onset Neuropsychiatric Syndrome: An Observational Study of Patients Followed by an Academic Community-Based Pediatric Acute-Onset Neuropsychiatric Syndrome Clinic. Journal of Child and Adolescent Psychopharmacology, 27(7), 619–628. https://doi.org/10.1089/cap.2016.0193

21 Paluck, E., Katzenstein, D., Frankish, C. J., Herbert, C. P., Milner, R., Speert, D., & Chambers, K. (2001). Prescribing practices and attitudes toward giving children antibiotics. Canadian family physician Medecin mde famille canadien, 47, 521–527.

22 Gerentes, M., Pelissolo, A., Rajagopal, K., Tamouza, R., & Hamdani, N. (2019). Obsessive-Compulsive Disorder: Autoimmunity and Neuroinflammation. Current Psychiatry Reports, 21(8), 78. https://doi.org/10.1007/s11920-019-1062-8

23 Orefici, G., Cardona, F., Cox, C. J., & Cunningham, M.W. (2016). Pediatric Autoimmune Neuropsychiatric Disorders Associated with Streptococcal Infections (PANDAS). In: Ferretti JJ, Stevens DL, Fischetti VA, editors. Streptococcus pyogenes Basic Biology to Clinical Manifestations (2016). https://www.ncbi.nlm.nih.gov/books/NBK333433/

24 Orlovska, S., Vestergaard, C. H., Bech, B. H., Nordentoft, M., Vestergaard, M., & Benros, M. E. (2017). Association of Streptococcal Throat Infection With Mental Disorders: Testing Key Aspects of the PANDAS Hypothesis in a Nationwide Study. JAMA Psychiatry, 74 (7), 740–746. https://doi.org/10.1001/jamapsychiatry.2017.0995

25 Xu, J, et al. (2020). Antibodies From Children With PANDAS Bind Specifically to Striatal Cholinergic Interneurons and Alter Their Activity. Am Jrnl of Psychiatry 16 Jun 2020 https://doi.org/10.1176/appi.ajp.2020.19070698

The Introduction of PANS

26 Swedo, S. E., Leonard, H. L., Garvey, M., Mittleman, B., Allen, A. J., Perlmutter, S., Lougee, L., Dow, S., Zamkoff, J., & Dubbert, B. K. (1998). Pediatric autoimmune neuropsychiatric disorders associated with Streptococcal infections: clinical description of the first 50 cases. The American Journal of Psychiatry, 155(2), 264–271. https://doi.org/10.1176/ajp.155.2.264

27 Swedo, S. E., Leckman, J. F., Rose, N. R. (2012). From Research Subgroup to Clinical Syndrome: Modifying the PANDAS Criteria to Describe PANS (Pediatric Acute-onset Neuropsychiatric Syndrome). Pediatr Therapeut 2:113, 2012.

28 Tonsillectomy. PPN. (2020, September 10). Retrieved September 28, 2021, from www.pandasppn.org/tonsillectomy

29 Prasad, N, et al. (2021). Role of tonsillectomy and adenoidectomy in parental satisfaction of treatments for PANDAS. American Journal of Otolaryngology, 2021, 102963, ISSN 0196-0709, DOI: 10.1016/j.amjoto.2021.102963.

30 Demesh, D, Virbalas, JM, Bent, JP. (2015). The Role of Tonsillectomy in the Treatment of Pediatric Autoimmune Neuropsychiatric Disorders Associated With Streptococcal Infections (PANDAS). JAMA Otolaryngol Head Neck Surg. 2015; 141(3): 272–275. doi:10.1001/jamaoto.2014.3407

31 Pavone, P, Rapisarda, V, Serra, A, et al. (2018). Pediatric autoimmune neuropsychiatry disorder associated with group a Streptococcal infection: The role of surgical treatment. International Journal of Immunopathology and Pharmacology, vol. 27, no. 3, 371–378

32 Alexander, Z, et al. (2011). Pediatric autoimmune neuropsychiatric disorders associated with Streptococcal infections (PANDAS): An indication for tonsillectomy. International Journal of Pediatric Otorhinolaryngology, vol. 75, no. 6, 872-873, 2011.

33 Heubi, et al. (2003). PANDAS: Pediatric autoimmune neuropsychiatric disorders associated with Streptococcal infections An uncommon, but important indication for tonsillectomy. International Journal of Pediatric Otorhinolaryngology, vol. 67, no. 8, 837–840, 2003.

34 Murphy, TK, et al. (2013). Tonsillectomies and adenoidectomies do not prevent the onset of pediatric autoimmune neuropsychiatric disorder associated with group a Streptococcus. The Pediatric Infectious Disease Journal, vol. 32, no. 8, 834–838, 2013.

35 Melamed, I, et al. (2020). Benefits of IVIG in Pediatric Acute-Onset Neuropsychiatric Syndrome. Neurology April 2020, 94 (15 Supplement) 2411

36 Latimer, ME, et al. (2015). Therapeutic Plasma Apheresis as a Treatment for 35 Severely Ill Children and Adolescents with Pediatric Autoimmune Neuropsychiatric Disorders Associated with Streptococcal Infections. Journal of Child and Adolescent Psychopharmacology. Feb 2015.70-75.http://doi.org/10.1089/cap.2014.008

37 Grassi, G, Cecchelli, C, Vignozzi, L, Pacini, S. (2021). Investigational and Experimental Drugs to Treat Obsessive-Compulsive Disorder. J Exp Pharmacol. 2021; 12: 695-706. Published 2021 Jan 5. doi:10.2147/JEP.S255375

Meet the Infectious Agents

Group A Streptococcus and PANDAS

38 Swedo, SE, Leonard, HL, Garvey, M, et al. (1998). Pediatric autoimmune neuropsychiatric disorders associated with Streptococcal infections: clinical description of the first 50 cases. Am. J. Psychiatry. 155(2), 264-271.

39 Brimberg, L, Benhar, I, Mascaro-Blanco, A, et al. (2012). Behavioral, pharmacological, and immunological abnormalities after Streptococcal exposure: a novel rat model of Sydenham chorea and related neuropsychiatric disorders. Neuropsychopharmacology. 2012; 37(9): 2076-2087.

40 Johansson, L, et al. (2010). Getting under the Skin: The Immunopathogenesis of Streptococcus pyogenes Deep Tissue Infections. Clinical Infectious Diseases, Volume 51, Issue 1, 1 July 2010, 58–65, https://doi.org/10.1086/653116.

41 Dafna, L, et al. (2014). Behavioral and neural effects of intra-striatal infusion of anti-Streptococcal antibodies in rats. Brain, Behavior, and Immunity. Volume 38, 2014, 249-262, https://doi.org/10.1016/j.bbi.2014.02.009.

42 van Toorn, D, et al. (2004). Distinguishing PANDAS from Sydenham's chorea: case report and review of the literature. European Journal of Paediatric Neurology. Volume 8, Issue 4, 2004, 211-216, https://doi.org/10.1016/j.ejpn.2004.03.005

43 Guilherme, L, et al. (2006). Molecular mimicry in the autoimmune pathogenesis of rheumatic heart disease. Autoimmunity, 39:1, 31-39, DOI: 10.1080/08916930500484674

44 Chang, K., Frankovich, J., Cooperstock, M., Cunningham, M. W., Latimer, M. E., Murphy, T. K., Pasternack, M., Thienemann, M., Williams, K., Walter, J., Swedo, S. E., & PANS Collaborative Consortium. (2015). Clinical evaluation of youth with pediatric acute-onset neuropsychiatric syndrome (PANS): recommendations from the 2013 PANS Consensus Conference. Journal of Child and Adolescent Psychopharmacology, 25(1), 3–13. https://doi.org/10.1089/cap.2014.0084

45 Prato, A, et al. (2021) Diagnostic Approach to Pediatric Autoimmune Neuropsychiatric Disorders Associated With Streptococcal Infections (PANDAS): A Narrative Review of Literature Data. Frontiers in Pediatrics, Volume 9. 10.3389/fped.2021.746639

46 Kaplan, EL, et al. (1998). AntiStreptolysin O and anti-deoxyribonuclease B titers: normal values for children ages 2 to 12 in the United States. Pediatrics, vol. 101, no. 1, part 1, 86–88, 1998.

47 Blyth, CC, et al. (2006). Anti-Streptococcal antibodies in the diagnosis of acute and postStreptococcal disease: Streptokinase versus Streptolysin O and deoxyribonuclease B. Pathology, Volume 38, Issue 2, 2006, 152-156, https://doi.org/10.1080/00313020600557060.

48 Kiessling, L. S., Marcotte, A. C., & Culpepper, L. (1993). Antineuronal antibodies in movement disorders. Pediatrics, 92(1), 39–43.

49 Cox, C, et al. (2015). Antineuronal Antibodies in a Heterogeneous Group of Youth and Young Adults with Tics and Obsessive-Compulsive Disorder. Journal of Child and Adolescent Psychopharmacology, Feb 2015. 76-85, http://doi.org/10.1089/cap.2014.0048

50 Chain, J, et al. (2020). Autoantibody Biomarkers for Basal Ganglia Encephalitis in Sydenham Chorea and Pediatric Autoimmune Neuropsychiatric Disorder Associated With Streptococcal Infections. Frontiers in Psychiatry. VOLUME 11. 10.3389/fpsyt.2020.00564

51 Kalra, M. G., Higgins, K. E., & Perez, E. D. (2016). Common Questions About Streptococcal Pharyngitis. American Family Physician, 94(1), 24–31.

Mycoplasma and PANS

52 Swedo, E.A., Leckman, J.F., & Rose, N.R. (2012). From Research Subgroup to Clinical Syndrome: Modifying the PANDAS Criteria to Describe PANS Pediatric Acute-onset Neuropsychiatric. Pediatrics & Therapeutics, 2, 1-8.

53 National Center for Immunization and Respiratory Diseases (2017) Mycoplasma pneumonia Infection [Fact Sheet]. Center for Disease Control and Prevention www.cdc.gov/pneumonia/atypical/Mycoplasma/downloads/Mycoplasma-Fact-Sheet-2017.pdf

54 Chang, K., Frankovich, J., Cooperstock, M., Cunningham, M. W., Latimer, M. E., Murphy, T. K., Pasternack, M., Thienemann, M., Williams, K., Walter, J., Swedo, S. E., & PANS Collaborative Consortium. (2015). Clinical evaluation of youth with pediatric acute-onset neuropsychiatric syndrome (PANS): recommendations from the 2013 PANS Consensus Conference. Journal of Child and Adolescent Psychopharmacology, 25(1), 3–13. https://doi.org/10.1089/cap.2014.0084

55 Thurman, K. A., Walter, N. D., Schwartz, S. B., Mitchell, S. L., Dillon, M. T., Baughman, A. L., Deutscher, M., Fulton, J. P., Tongren, J. E., Hicks, L. A., & Winchell, J. M. (2009). Comparison of laboratory diagnostic procedures for detection of Mycoplasma pneumoniae in community outbreaks. Clinical infectious diseases an official publication of the Infectious Diseases Society of America, 48(9), 1244–1249. https://doi.org/10.1086/597775

56 Schnell, J, et al. (2022) Mycoplasma pneumoniae IgG positivity is associated with tic severity in chronic tic disorders. Brain, Behavior, and Immunity (99) 281-288. ISSN 0889-1591, https://doi.org/10.1016/j.bbi.2021.10.012.

57 Leal, S, Totten, A, Xiao, L, et al. (2020). Evaluation of Commercial Molecular Diagnostic Methods for the Detection and Determination of Macrolide Resistance in Mycoplasma pneumoniae. J Clin Microbiol. 2020; doi:10.1128/JCM.00242-20.

58 Ansah, C., & Mensah, K. B. (2013). A review of the anticancer potential of the antimalarial herbal cryptolepis sanguinolenta and its major alkaloid cryptolepine. Ghana Medical Journal, 47(3), 137–147.

59 McCarthy, E., & O'Mahony, J. M. (2011). What's in a Name? Can Mullein Weed Beat TB Where Modern Drugs Are Failing?. Evidence-Based Complementary and Alternative medicine eCAM, 2011, 239237. https://doi.org/10.1155/2011/239237

60 Arjoon, A. V., Saylor, C. V., & May, M. (2012). In Vitro efficacy of antimicrobial extracts against the atypical ruminant pathogen Mycoplasma mycoides subsp. capri. BMC Complementary and Alternative Medicine, 12, 169. https://doi.org/10.1186/1472-6882-12-169

61 Neag, M. A., Mocan, A., Echeverría, J., Pop, R. M., Bocsan, C. I., Crişan, G., & Buzoianu, A. D. (2018). Berberine: Botanical Occurrence, Traditional Uses, Extraction Methods, and Relevance in Cardiovascular, Metabolic, Hepatic, and Renal Disorders. Frontiers in Pharmacology, 9, 557. https://doi.org/10.3389/fphar.2018.00557

62 Sekita, Y., Murakami, K., Yumoto, H., Amoh, T., Fujiwara, N., Ogata, S., Matsuo, T., Miyake, Y., & Kashiwada, Y. (2016). Preventive Effects of Houttuynia cordata Extract for Oral Infectious Diseases. BioMed Research International, 2016, 2581876. https://doi.org/10.1155/2016/2581876

63 Nicolson, G. L. (2019). Pathogenic Mycoplasma infections in chronic illnesses: General considerations in selecting conventional and integrative treatments. International Journal of Clinical Medicine, 10(10), 477–522. https://doi.org/10.4236/ijcm.2019.1010041.

Viruses

64 Caroff, S. N., Jain, R., & Morley, J. F. (2020). Revisiting amantadine as a treatment for drug-induced movement disorders. Annals of Clinical Psychiatry official journal of the American Academy of Clinical Psychiatrists, 32(3), 198–208.

65 Joseph T. Giacino JT et al. Placebo-Controlled Trial of Amantadine for Severe Traumatic Brain Injury. N Engl J Med 2012; 366: 819-826. DOI:10.1056/NEJMoa1102609

66 Araújo, R., Aranda-Martínez, J. D., & Aranda-Abreu, G. E. (2020). Amantadine Treatment for People with COVID-19. Archives of medical research, 51(7), 739–740. https://doi.org/10.1016/j.arcmed.2020.06.009

67 Morrow, K., Choi, S., Young, K., Haidar, M., Boduch, C., & Bourgeois, J. A. (2021). Amantadine for the treatment of childhood and adolescent psychiatric symptoms. Proceedings (Baylor University. Medical Center), 34(5), 566–570. https://doi.org/10.1080/08998280.2021.1925827

68 Patel, S., & Vajdy, M. (2015). Induction of cellular and molecular immunomodulatory pathways by vitamin A and flavonoids. Expert opinion on biological therapy, 15(10), 1411–1428. https://doi.org/10.1517/14712598.2015.1066331

69 Mousavi, S., Bereswill, S., & Heimesaat, M. M. (2019). Immunomodulatory and Antimicrobial Effects of Vitamin C. European Journal of Microbiology & Immunology, 9(3), 73–79. https://doi.org/10.1556/1886.2019.00016

70 Siddiqui, M., Manansala, J. S., Abdulrahman, H. A., Nasrallah, G. K., Smatti, M. K., Younes, N., Althani, A. A., & Yassine, H. M. (2020). Immune Modulatory Effects of Vitamin D on Viral Infections. Nutrients, 12(9), 2879. https://doi.org/10.3390/nu12092879

71 Read, S. A., Obeid, S., Ahlenstiel, C., & Ahlenstiel, G. (2019). The Role of Zinc in Antiviral Immunity. Advances in nutrition (Bethesda, Md.), 10(4), 696–710. https://doi.org/10.1093/advances/nmz013

72 Ferren, M., Horvat, B., & Mathieu, C. (2019). Measles Encephalitis: Towards New Therapeutics. Viruses, 11(11), 1017. https://doi.org/10.3390/v11111017

73 Cutrona, K. J., Kaufman, B. A., Figueroa, D. M., & Elmore, D. E. (2015). Role of arginine and lysine in the antimicrobial mechanism of histone-derived antimicrobial peptides. FEBS letters, 589(24 Pt B), 3915–3920. https://doi.org/10.1016/j.febslet.2015.11.002

74 Barker, L. A., Bakkum, B. W., & Chapman, C. (2019). The Clinical Use of Monolaurin as a Dietary Supplement: A Review of the Literature. Journal of Chiropractic Medicine, 18(4), 305–310. https://doi.org/10.1016/j.jcm.2019.02.004

75 Kallon, S., Li, X., Ji, J., Chen, C., Xi, Q., Chang, S., Xue, C., Ma, J., Xie, Q., & Zhang, Y. (2013). Astragalus polysaccharide enhances immunity and inhibits H9N2 avian influenza virus in vitro and in vivo. Journal of Animal Science and Biotechnology, 4(1), 22. https://doi.org/10.1186/2049-1891-4-22

76 Hossain, S., Urbi, Z., Karuniawati, H., Mohiuddin, R. B., Moh Qrimida, A., Allzrag, A., Ming, L. C., Pagano, E., & Capasso, R. (2021). Andrographis paniculata (Burm. f.) Wall. ex Nees: An Updated Review of Phytochemistry, Antimicrobial Pharmacology, and Clinical Safety and Efficacy. Life (Basel, Switzerland), 11(4), 348. https://doi.org/10.3390/life11040348

77 Warowicka, A., Nawrot, R., & Goździcka-Józefiak, A. (2020). Antiviral activity of berberine. Archives of Virology, 165(9), 1935–1945. https://doi.org/10.1007/s00705-020-04706-3

78 Krawitz, C., Mraheil, M. A., Stein, M., Imirzalioglu, C., Domann, E., Pleschka, S., & Hain, T. (2011). Inhibitory activity of a standardized elderberry liquid extract against clinically-relevant human respiratory bacterial pathogens and influenza A and B viruses. BMC Complementary and Alternative Medicine, 11, 16. https://doi.org/10.1186/1472-6882-11-16

79 Ben-Amor, I., Musarra-Pizzo, M., Smeriglio, A., D'Arrigo, M., Pennisi, R., Attia, H., Gargouri, B., Trombetta, D., Mandalari, G., & Sciortino, M. T. (2021). Phytochemical Characterization of Olea europea Leaf Extracts and Assessment of Their Anti-Microbial and Anti-HSV-1 Activity. Viruses, 13(6), 1085. https://doi.org/10.3390/v13061085

80 Hasan, M. K., Ara, I., Mondal, M., & Kabir, Y. (2021). Phytochemistry, pharmacological activity, and potential health benefits of Glycyrrhiza glabra. Heliyon, 7(6), e07240. https://doi.org/10.1016/j.heliyon.2021.e07240

81 Miraj, S., Rafieian-Kopaei, & Kiani, S. (2017). Melissa officinalis L: A Review Study With an Antioxidant Prospective. Journal of Evidence-Based Complementary & Alternative Medicine, 22(3), 385–394. https://doi.org/10.1177/2156587216663433

82 Researched Nutritionals. (2021, July 15). A Guide to Transfer Factors and Immune System Health, by Aaron White, Ph.D. https://www.researchednutritionals.com/product/transfer-factor-book-a-guide-to-transfer-factors-and-immune-system-health

83 Krishnamoorthy, N, Abdulnour, R-EE, Walker, KH, Engstrom, BD, Levy, BD. (2018). Specialized proresolving mediators in innate and adaptive immune responses in airway diseases. Physiol Rev. 2018; 98: 1335–1370.

84 Nezgovorova, V, et al. (2021) Modulating neuroinflammation in COVID-19 patients with obsessive-compulsive disorder, Journal of Psychiatric Research. ISSN 0022-3956. https://doi.org/10.1016/j.jpsychires.2021.11.025.

Yeast Dysbiosis

85 Appleton, J. (2018). The Gut-Brain Axis: Influence of Microbiota on Mood and Mental Health. Integrative Medicine (Encinitas, Calif.), 17(4), 28–32

86 Rogers, G., Keating, D., Young, R. et al. (2016). From gut dysbiosis to altered brain function and mental illness: mechanisms and pathways. Mol Psychiatry 21, 738–748. https://doi.org/10.1038/mp.2016.50

87 Foster, J. A., & McVey Neufeld, K. A. (2013). Gut-brain axis: how the microbiome influences anxiety and depression. Trends in neurosciences, 36(5), 305–312. https://doi.org/10.1016/j.tins.2013.01.005

88 Quagliariello, A., Del Chierico, F., Russo, A., Reddel, S., Conte, G., Lopetuso, L. R., Ianiro, G., Dallapiccola, B., Cardona, F., Gasbarrini, A., & Putignani, L. (2018). Gut Microbiota Profiling and Gut-Brain Crosstalk in Children Affected by Pediatric Acute-Onset Neuropsychiatric Syndrome and Pediatric Autoimmune Neuropsychiatric Disorders Associated With Streptococcal Infections. Frontiers in Microbiology, 9, 675. https://doi.org/10.3389/fmicb.2018.00675

89 Aggarwal, N, Bhateja, S, Arora, G, Yasmin, T. (2018). Candidiasis- The Most Common Fungal Infection of Oral Cavity. Biomedical Journal of Scientific and Technical Research, 8(3): 6487-6491.

90 Haruta, S, Kanno, N. (2015). Survivability of microbes in natural environments and their ecological impacts. Microbes and Environment, 30(2): 123-125.

91 McKenzie, CG, Koser, U, Lewis, LE, Bain, JM, Mora-Montes, HM, Barker ,RN, Gow, NA, Erwig, LP. (2010). Contribution of Candida albicans cell wall components to recognition by and escape from murine macrophages. Infection and Immunity, 78(4):1650-1658.

92 Crook, William. (1985). The Yeast Connection: A Medical Breakthrough. Knopf Doubleday Publishing Group.

93 Alberti, A., Corbella, S., Taschieri, S., Francetti, L., Fakhruddin, K. S., & Samaranayake, L. P. (2021). Fungal species in endodontic infections: A systematic review and meta-analysis. PloS one, 16(7), e0255003. https://doi.org/10.1371/journal.pone.0255003

94 Mayer, F. L., Wilson, D., & Hube, B. (2013). Candida albicans pathogenicity mechanisms. Virulence, 4(2), 119–128. https://doi.org/10.4161/viru.22913

95 Carding S, et al. (2015). Dysbiosis of the gut microbiota in disease. Microbial Ecology in Health and Disease. 2015; 26(1), 26191.

96 Shaw, W, et al. (2000). Assessment of Antifungal Drug Therapy in Autism by Measurement of Suspected Microbial Metabolites in Urine with Gas Chromatography-Mass Spectrometry. Clinical Practice of Alternative Medicine 1(1): 15-26, 2000

97 Wong, B, Brauer, K, Clemens, J, Beggs, S. (1990). Effects of gastrointestinal Candidiasis, antibiotics, dietary arabinitol, and cortisone acetate on levels of the Candida metabolite D-arabinitol in rat serum and urine. Infect Immunol. 1990;58:283-288.

98 Qin, J., Yang, H., Shan, Z., Jiang, L., & Zhang, Q. (2021). Clinical efficacy and safety of antifungal drugs for the treatment of Candida parapsilosis infections: a systematic review and network meta-analysis. Journal of Medical Microbiology, 70(10), 001434. https://doi.org/10.1099/jmm.0.001434

99 Spampinato, C., & Leonardi, D. (2013). Candida infections, causes, targets, and resistance mechanisms: traditional and alternative antifungal agents. BioMed Research International, 2013, 204237. https://doi.org/10.1155/2013/204237

100 Černáková, L., Roudbary, M., Brás, S., Tafaj, S., & Rodrigues, C. F. (2021). Candida auris: A Quick Review on Identification, Current Treatments, and Challenges. International Journal of Molecular Sciences, 22(9), 4470. https://doi.org/10.3390/ijms22094470

101 Lu, M., Dai, T., Murray, C. K., & Wu, M. X. (2018). Bactericidal Property of Oregano Oil Against Multidrug-Resistant Clinical Isolates. Frontiers in Microbiology, 9, 2329. https://doi.org/10.3389/fmicb.2018.02329

102 Tsutsumi-Arai, C., Takakusaki, K., Arai, Y., Terada-Ito, C., Takebe, Y., Imamura, T., Ide, S., Tatehara, S., Tokuyama-Toda, R., Wakabayashi, N., & Satomura, K. (2019). Grapefruit seed extract effectively inhibits the Candida albicans biofilms development on polymethyl methacrylate denture-base resin. PloS one, 14(5), e0217496. https://doi.org/10.1371/journal.pone.0217496

103 Omura, Y., O'Young, B., Jones, M., Pallos, A., Duvvi, H., & Shimotsuura, Y. (2011). Caprylic acid in the effective treatment of intractable medical problems of frequent urination, incontinence, chronic upper respiratory infection, root canalled tooth infection, ALS, etc., caused by asbestos & mixed infections of Candida albicans, Helicobacter pylori & Cytomegalovirus with or without other microorganisms & mercury. Acupuncture & Electro-Therapeutics Research, 36(1-2), 19–64. https://doi.org/10.3727/036012911803860886

104 Hofling, J., et al. (2010). Antimicrobial potential of some plant extracts against Candida species. Braz J Biol. 2010 Nov; 70(4): 1065-8.

105 Melo e Silva, F., et al. (2009). Evaluation of the antifungal potential of Brazilian Cerrado medicinal plants." Mycoses. 52(6): 511-7.

106 Imenshahidi, M., & Hosseinzadeh, H. (2019). Berberine and barberry (Berberis vulgaris): A clinical review. Phytotherapy research: PTR, 33(3), 504–523. https://doi.org/10.1002/ptr.6252

107 Proškovcová, M., Čonková, E., Váczi, P., Harčárová, M., & Malinovská, Z. (2021). Antibiofilm activity of selected plant essential oils from the Lamiaceae family against Candida albicans clinical isolates. Annals of Agricultural and Environmental Medicine: AAEM, 28(2), 260–266. https://doi.org/10.26444/aaem/135892

108 Borlinghaus, J., Albrecht, F., Gruhlke, M. C., Nwachukwu, I. D., & Slusarenko, A. J. (2014). Allicin: chemistry and biological properties. Molecules (Basel, Switzerland), 19(8), 12591–12618. https://doi.org/10.3390/molecules190812591

109 Yamaguchi H. (1974). Mycelial development and chemical alteration of Candida albicans from biotin insufficiency. Sabouraudia, 12(3), 320–328.

110 Okamoto-Shibayama, K., Yoshida, A., & Ishihara, K. (2021). Inhibitory Effect of Resveratrol on Candida albicans Biofilm Formation. The Bulletin of Tokyo Dental College, 62(1), 1–6. https://doi.org/10.2209/tdcpublication.2020-0023

111 Afrin, S., Promee, J. S., Nahid, M., Satter, M. A., Haque, M. A., Sarker, A. K. & Bhuiyan, M. N. I. (2021). Influence of thermal and osmotic pressure on the growth and viability of Candida shehatae var shehatae. Journal of Yeast and Fungal Research 12(2), 20-27.

112 Cavalheiro, M., & Teixeira, M. C. (2018). Candida Biofilms: Threats, Challenges, and Promising Strategies. Frontiers in Medicine, 5, 28. https://doi.org/10.3389/fmed.2018.00028

113 Shichiri-Negoro, Y, Tsutsumi-Arai, C, Arai, Y, Satomura, K, Arakawa, S, Wakabayashi, N. (2021). Ozone ultrafine bubble water inhibits the early formation of Candida albicans biofilms. PLoS One. 2021 Dec 10; 16(12): e0261180. doi: 10.1371/journal.pone.0261180.

114 Homei, A, Worboys, M. (2013). Fungal Disease in Britain and the United States 1850–2000: Mycoses and Modernity. Basingstoke (UK): Palgrave Macmillan, Chapter 3, Candida: A Disease of Antibiotics. Available from: www.ncbi.nlm.nih.gov/books/NBK169215/

Mold and Chronic Inflammatory Response Syndrome (CIRS)

115 McMahon, SW, Shoemaker, RC, Ryan, JC. (2016). Reduction in Forebrain Parenchymal and Cortical Grey Matter Swelling across Treatment Groups in Patients with Inflammatory Illness Acquired Following Exposure to Water- Damaged Buildings. Journal of Neuroscience and Clinical Research. 2016; 1:1.

116 Shoemaker, R, Maizel, M. (2008). Innate immunity, MR spectroscopy, HLA DR, TGF beta-1, VIP and capillary hypoperfusion define acute and chronic human illness acquired following exposure to water-damaged buildings. International Healthy Buildings.

117 Doi, K & Uetsuka, K. (2011). Mechanisms of mycotoxin-induced neurotoxicity through oxidative stress-associated pathways. Int J Mol Sci 12, 5213-5237.

118 Shoemaker, RC. (1998) Treatment of persistent Pfiesteria-human illness syndrome. Maryland Medical Journal; 47: 64-66.

119 Shoemaker, RC & Lawson, W. (2007). Pfiesteria in Estuarine Waters: The question of health risks. Environmental Health Perspectives; 115: A2-A3.

120 Shoemaker, RC, Mark, L, McMahon, S, Thrasher, J, Grimes, C. (2010). Research committee report on diagnosis and treatment of chronic inflammatory response syndrome caused by exposure to the interior environment of water-damaged buildings. Policyholders of America. 2010 July 27: 1-161.

121 De Santis, B1, Brera, C, Mezzelani, A, et al. (2017). Role of mycotoxins in the pathobiology of autism: A first evidence. Nutr Neurosci 2017 Aug 10:1-13. doi: 10.1080/1028415X.2017.1357793

122 Guilford, F. T. & Hope, J. (2014). Deficient glutathione in the pathophysiology of mycotoxin-related illness. Toxins (Basel) 2014, 6, 608-623.

123 McMahon, S.W., Kundomal, K.A., & Yangalasetty, S. (2017). Pediatrics Norms for Visual Contrast Sensitivity Using an APT VCS Tester. Medical research archives, 5.

124 Shoemaker, RC, House, D, Ryan, JC. (2014). Structural brain abnormalities in patients with inflammatory illness acquired following exposure to water-damaged buildings: a volumetric MRI study using NeuroQuant®. Neurotoxicology and Teratology. 2014 Sep-Oct;45: 18-26.

125 Shoemaker, RC, House, D, Ryan, J. (2010). Defining the neurotoxin derived illness chronic ciguatera using markers of chronic systemic inflammatory disturbances: A case/control study. Neurotoxicology and Teratology 2010; 633-639.

126 Lichtenstein, R, et al. (2015). Environmental mold and mycotoxin exposures elicit specific cytokine and chemokine responses. PloS one, 10(5), e0126926. https://doi.org/10.1371/journal.pone.0126926

127 Brewer, J. H., Thrasher, J. D., & Hooper, D. (2013). Chronic illness associated with mold and mycotoxins: is naso-sinus fungal biofilm the culprit?. Toxins, 6(1), 66–80. https://doi.org/10.3390/toxins6010066

128 Berndtson, K, McMahon, S, Ackerley, M, Rapaport, S, Gupta, S, Shoemaker, RC. (2015). Medically sound investigation and remediation of water-damaged buildings in cases of CIRS-WDB: Consensus Statement Part 1. Center for Research on Biotoxin Associated Illness. 2015.

129 Shoemaker, RC & Hudnell, D. (2004). A time-series study of sick building syndrome: chronic, biotoxin-associated illness from exposure to water-damaged buildings. Neurotoxicology and Teratology 2004; 1-18.

Other Infections: Parasites, Clostridia, Lyme Disease, and Co-infections

130 www.cdc.gov/parasites/references_resources/diagnosis.html

131 Campbell, S, Soman-Faulkner, K. (2022). Antiparasitic Drugs. [Updated 2021 Sep 8]. In: StatPearls [Internet]. Treasure Island (FL): StatPearls Publishing; 2022 Jan. Available from: www.ncbi.nlm.nih.gov/books/NBK544251/

132 Dahl, W. J., & Stewart, M. L. (2015). Position of the Academy of Nutrition and Dietetics: Health Implications of Dietary Fiber. Journal of the Academy of Nutrition and Dietetics, 115(11), 1861–1870. https://doi.org/10.1016/j.jand.2015.09.003

133 Robinson, R. D., Williams, L. A., Lindo, J. F., Terry, S. I., & Mansingh, A. (1990). Inactivation of strongyloides stercoralis filariform larvae in vitro by six Jamaican plant extracts and three commercial anthelmintics. The West Indian medical journal, 39(4), 213–217.

134 Beshay, E. (2018). Therapeutic efficacy of Artemisia absinthium against Hymenolepis nana: in vitro and in vivo studies in comparison with the anthelmintic praziquantel. Journal of Helminthology, 92(3), 298–308. https://doi.org/10.1017/S0022149X17000529

135 Jahanban-Esfahlan, A., Ostadrahimi, A., Tabibiazar, M., & Amarowicz, R. (2019). A Comprehensive Review on the Chemical Constituents and Functional Uses of Walnut (Juglans spp.) Husk. International Journal of Molecular Sciences, 20(16), 3920. https://doi.org/10.3390/ijms20163920

136 Czepiel, J., Dróżdż, M., Pituch, H., Kuijper, E. J., Perucki, W., Mielimonka, A., Goldman, S., Wultańska, D., Garlicki, A., & Biesiada, G. (2019). Clostridium difficile infection: review. European journal of clinical microbiology & infectious diseases official publication of the European Society of Clinical Microbiology, 38(7), 1211–1221. https://doi.org/10.1007/s10096-019-03539-6

137 Macfabe, D. F. (2012). Short-chain fatty acid fermentation products of the gut microbiome: implications in autism spectrum disorders. Microbial Ecology in Health and Disease, 23, 10.3402/mehd.v23i0.19260. https://doi.org/10.3402/mehd.v23i0.19260

138 Shaw, W. (2010). Increased urinary excretion of a 3-(3-hydroxyphenyl)-3-hydroxypropionic acid (HPHPA), an abnormal phenylalanine metabolite of Clostridia spp. in the gastrointestinal tract, in urine samples from patients with autism and schizophrenia. Nutritional Neuroscience; 13(3): 135-143.

139 Persico, AM, et. al. (2012). Urinary p-cresol in autism spectrum disorders, Neurotoxicol Teratol. 2013 Mar-Apr; 36: 82-90, 2012 Sep 10.

140 Nelson, R. L., Suda, K. J., & Evans, C. T. (2017). Antibiotic treatment for Clostridium difficile-associated diarrhoea in adults. The Cochrane database of systematic reviews, 3(3), CD004610. https://doi.org/10.1002/14651858.CD004610.pub5

141 Lv, Z., Peng, G., Liu, W., Xu, H., & Su, J. (2015). Berberine blocks the relapse of Clostridium difficile infection in C57BL/6 mice after standard vancomycin treatment. Antimicrobial agents and chemotherapy, 59(7), 3726–3735. https://doi.org/10.1128/AAC.04794-14

142 Aljarallah, KM. (2016). Inhibition of Clostridium difficile by natural herbal extracts, Journal of Taibah University Medical Sciences. http://dx.doi.org/10.1016/j.jtumed.2016.05.006

143 De Wolfe, TJ, Eggers, S, Barker, AK, Kates, AE, Dill-McFarland, KA, Suen, G, et al. (2018). Oral probiotic combination of Lactobacillus and Bifidobacterium alters the gastrointestinal microbiota during antibiotic treatment for Clostridium difficile infection. PLoS ONE 13(9): e0204253. https://doi.org/10.1371/journal.pone.0204253

144 https://www.cdc.gov/lyme/treatment/NeurologicLyme.html

145 Richter, D., Spielman, A., Komar, N., & Matuschka, F. (2000). Competence of American Robins as Reservoir Hosts for Lyme Disease Spirochetes. Emerging Infectious Diseases, 6(2), 133-138. https://doi.org/10.3201/eid0602.000205.

146 Piesman, J., Mather, T. N., Sinsky, R. J., & Spielman, A. (1987). Duration of tick attachment and Borrelia burgdorferi transmission. Journal of Clinical Microbiology, 25(3), 557–558. https://doi.org/10.1128/jcm.25.3.557-558.1987

147 Eisen, L. (2018). Pathogen transmission in relation to duration of attachment by Ixodes scapularis ticks. Ticks and tick-borne diseases, 9(3), 535–542. https://doi.org/10.1016/j.ttbdis.2018.01.002

148 Leeflang, MM, Ang, CW, Berkhout, J, Bijlmer, HA, Van Bortel, W, Brandenburg, AH, Van Burgel. ND, Van Dam. AP, Dessau, RB, Fingerle, V, Hovius, JW, Jaulhac, B, Meijer, B, Van Pelt, W, Schellekens, JF, Spijker, R, Stelma, FF, Stanek, G, Verduyn-Lunel, F, Zeller. H, Sprong, H. (2016). The diagnostic accuracy of serological tests for Lyme borreliosis in Europe: a systematic review and meta-analysis. BMC Infect Dis. 2016 Mar 25;16:140. doi: 10.1186/s12879-016-1468-4.

149 Hatchette, T. F., Davis, I., & Johnston, B. L. (2014). Lyme disease: clinical diagnosis and treatment. Canada communicable disease report = Releve des maladies transmissibles au Canada, 40(11), 194–208. https://doi.org/10.14745/ccdr.v40i11a01

150 Schwameis, M, et al. (2017). Topical azithromycin for the prevention of Lyme borreliosis: a randomised, placebo-controlled, phase 3 efficacy trial. The Lancet Infectious Diseases, Volume 17, Issue 3, 2017, 322-329, https://doi.org/10.1016/S1473-3099(16)30529-1.

151 Stricker, R. B. (2007). Counterpoint: long-term antibiotic therapy improves persistent symptoms associated with lyme disease. Clinical infectious diseases an official publication of the Infectious Diseases Society of America, 45(2), 149–157. https://doi.org/10.1086/518853

152 Goc, A, et al. (2016). Cooperation of Doxycycline with Phytochemicals and Micronutrients Against Active and Persistent Forms of Borrelia sp. Int J Biol Sci. 2016 Jul 22. doi: 10.7150/ijbs.16060

153 Pound, MW & May, DB. (2005). Proposed mechanisms and preventative options of Jarisch-Herxheimer reactions. J Clin Pharm Ther 2005; 30: 291-295.

154 Forsgren, S., Nathan N., & Anderson, W. (2014). Mold and Mycotoxins: Often Overlooked Factors in Chronic Lyme Disease. Mold, Mycotoxins, Lyme; Townsend Letter for Doctors & Patients. Retrieved July 9, 2021, from www.townsendletter.com/July2014/mold0714.html

155 Stricker, R. B., Lautin, A., & Burrascano, J. J. (2005). Lyme disease: point/counterpoint. Expert review of anti-infective therapy, 3(2), 155-165. https://doi.org/10.1586/14787210.3.2.155

156 Feng, J, et al. (2020). Evaluation of Natural and Botanical Medicines for Activity Against Growing and Non-growing Forms of B. burgdorferi. Front. Med., 21 February 2020. DOI=10.3389/fmed.2020.00006

157 Adelson, ME, Rao, RV, Tilton, RC, Cabets, K, Eskow, E, Fein, L, Occi, JL, Mordechai, E. (2004). Prevalence of Borrelia burgdorferi, Bartonella spp., Babesia microti, and Anaplasma phagocytophila in Ixodes scapularis ticks collected in Northern New Jersey. J Clin Microbiol. 2004 Jun; 42(6): 2799-801. doi: 10.1128/JCM.42.6.2799-2801.2004.

158 Lashnits, E, Maggi, R, Jarskog, F, Bradley, J, Breitschwerdt, E, Frohlich, F. (2021). Schizophrenia and Bartonella spp. Infection: A Pilot Case-Control Study. Vector Borne Zoonotic Dis. 2021 Jun; 21(6): 413-421. doi: 10.1089/vbz.2020.2729.

159 Lins, KA, Drummond, MR, Velho, PENF. (2019). Cutaneous manifestations of bartonellosis. An Bras Dermatol. 2019 Sep-Oct; 94(5): 594-602. doi: 10.1016/j.abd.2019.09.024.

160 Diuk-Wasser, M, et al. (2016). Coinfection by Ixodes Tick-Borne Pathogens: Ecological, Epidemiological, and Clinical Consequences, Trends in Parasitology, Volume 32, Issue 1,2016, Pages 30-42, https://doi.org/10.1016/j.pt.2015.09.008.

161 Lacout, A, El Hajjam, M, Marcy, PY, Perronne, C. (2018). The Persistent Lyme Disease: "True Chronic Lyme Disease" rather than "Post-treatment Lyme Disease Syndrome". J Glob Infect Dis. 2018 Jul-Sep; 10(3): 170-171. doi: 10.4103/jgid.jgid_152_17.

162 Maloney, EL. (2009). The Need for Clinical Judgment in the Diagnosis and Treatment of Lyme Disease. J Am Phys Surgeons 2009; 14(3): 82-89

163 Fallon, BA, Levin, ES, Schweitzer, PJ, Hardesty, D. (2010). Inflammation and central nervous system Lyme disease. Neurobiol Dis. 2010 Mar; 37(3): 534-41.

164 Hinckley, A, Connolly, N, Meek, J, Johnson, B, et al. (2014). Lyme disease testing by large commercial laboratories in the United States. Clin Infect Dis. 2014; 59(5): 676-681.

165 Cameron, D, Maloney, E, Johnson, L. (2014). Evidence assessment and guideline recommendations in Lyme disease: the clinical management of known tick bites, erythema migrans rashes and persistent disease. Expert Rev Anti Infect Ther, 2014 Sep; 12(9): 1103-1135.

Step 1: Eradicate the Pathogen

About the Antimicrobials

166 Swedo, S. E., Frankovich, J., & Murphy, T. K. (2017). Overview of Treatment of Pediatric Acute-Onset Neuropsychiatric Syndrome. Journal of Child and Adolescent Psychopharmacology, 27(7), 562–565. https://doi.org/10.1089/cap.2017.0042.

167 Snider, L. A., Lougee, L., Slattery, M., Grant, P., & Swedo, S. E. (2005). Antibiotic Prophylaxis with Azithromycin or Penicillin for Childhood-Onset Neuropsychiatric Disorders. Biological Psychiatry, 57(7), 788–792. https://doi.org/10.1016/j.biopsych.2004.12.035.

168 Cooperstock, M.S., Swedo, S.E., Pasternack, M.S., Murphy, T.K. (2017). Clinical Management of Pediatric Acute-Onset Neuropsychiatric Syndrome: Part III-Treatment and Prevention of Infections. Journal of Child and Adolescent Psychopharmacology, 27(7), 594-606. http://doi.org/10.1089/cap.2016.0151.

169 Murphy, T. K., Brennan, E. M., Johnco, C., Parker-Athill, E. C., Miladinovic, B., Storch, E. A., & Lewin, A. B. (2017). A Double-Blind Randomized Placebo-Controlled Pilot Study of Azithromycin in Youth with Acute-Onset Obsessive-Compulsive Disorder. Journal of Child and Adolescent Psychopharmacology, 27(7), 640–651. https://doi.org/10.1089/cap.2016.0190.

170 Venditto, V. J., Haydar, D., Abdel-Latif, A., Gensel, J. C., Anstead, M. I., Pitts, M. G., Creameans, J., Kopper, T. J., Peng, C., & Feola, D. J. (2021). Immunomodulatory Effects of Azithromycin Revisited: Potential Applications to COVID-19. Frontiers in Immunology, 12, 574425. https://doi.org/10.3389/fimmu.2021.574425

171 Albert, R. K., Schuller, J. L., & COPD Clinical Research Network. (2014). Macrolide Antibiotics And The Risk Of Cardiac Arrhythmias. American Journal of Respiratory and Critical Care Medicine, 189(10), 1173–1180. https://doi.org/10.1164/rccm.201402-0385CI.

172 Tauber, S. C., & Nau, R. (2008). Immunomodulatory Properties of Antibiotics. Current Molecular Pharmacology, 1(1), 68–79.

173 Pradhan, S., Madke, B., Kabra, P., & Singh, A. L. (2016). Anti-inflammatory and Immunomodulatory Effects of Antibiotics and Their Use in Dermatology. Indian Journal of Dermatology, 61(5), 469–481. https://doi.org/10.4103/0019-5154.190105

174 Kawai, Y., Miyashita, N., Kubo, M., Akaike, H., Kato, A., Nishizawa, Y., Saito, A., Kondo, E., Teranishi, H., Ogita, S., Tanaka, T., Kawasaki, K., Nakano, T., Terada, K., & Ouchi, K. (2013). Therapeutic efficacy of macrolides, minocycline, and tosufloxacin against macrolide-resistant Mycoplasma Pneumoniae Pneumonia in Pediatric Patients. Antimicrobial Agents and Chemotherapy, 57(5), 2252–2258. https://doi.org/10.1128/AAC.00048-13

175 Di Pierro, F., Colombo, M., Zanvit, A., Risso, P., & Rottoli, A. S. (2014). Use of Streptococcus salivarius K12 in the prevention of Streptococcal and viral pharyngotonsillitis in children. Drug, Healthcare and Patient Safety, 6, 15–20. https://doi.org/10.2147/DHPS.S59665

176 Srivastava, P., Upreti, D. K., Dhole, T. N., Srivastava, A. K., & Nayak, M. T. (2013). Antimicrobial Property of Extracts of Indian Lichen against Human Pathogenic Bacteria. Interdisciplinary perspectives on infectious diseases, 2013, 709348. https://doi.org/10.1155/2013/709348

177 Tozatti, M. G., Ferreira, D. S., Flauzino, L. G., Moraes, T., Martins, C. H., Groppo, M., Andrade e Silva, M. L., Januário, A. H., Pauletti, P. M., & Cunhaa, W. R. (2016). Activity of the Lichen Usnea steineri and its Major Metabolites against Gram-positive, Multidrug-resistant Bacteria. Natural Product Communications, 11(4), 493–496.

178 Glatthaar-Saalmüller, B., Sacher, F., & Esperester, A. (2001). Antiviral activity of an extract derived from roots of Eleutherococcus senticosus. Antiviral Research, 50(3), 223–228. https://doi.org/10.1016/s0166-3542(01)00143-7

179 Peng, L., Kang, S., Yin, Z., Jia, R., Song, X., Li, L., Li, Z., Zou, Y., Liang, X., Li, L., He, C., Ye, G., Yin, L., Shi, F., Lv, C., & Jing, B. (2015). Antibacterial Activity and Mechanism of Berberine Against Streptococcus agalactiae. International Journal of Clinical and Experimental Pathology, 8(5), 5217–5223.

180 Bansal, V., Gupta, M., Bhaduri, T., Shaikh, S. A., Sayed, F. R., Bansal, V., & Agrawal, A. (2019). Assessment of Antimicrobial Effectiveness of Neem and Clove Extract Against Streptococcus mutans and Candida albicans: An In vitro Study. Nigerian medical journal: Journal of the Nigeria Medical Association, 60(6), 285–289. https://doi.org/10.4103/nmj.NMJ_20_19

181 Chava, V. R., Manjunath, S. M., Rajanikanth, A. V., & Sridevi, N. (2012). The Efficacy of Neem Extract on Four Microorganisms Responsible for Causing Dental Caries Viz Streptococcus mutans, Streptococcus salivarius, Streptococcus mitis and Streptococcus sanguis: An In Vitro Study. The Journal of Contemporary Dental Practice, 13(6), 769–772. https://doi.org/10.5005/jp-journals-10024-1227.

182 Ghafari, O., Sharifi, A., Ahmadi, A., & Nayeri Fasaei, B. (2018). Antibacterial and anti-PmrA activity of plant essential oils against fluoroquinolone-resistant Streptococcus pneumoniae clinical isolates. Letters in Applied Microbiology, 67(6), 564–569. https://doi.org/10.1111/lam.13050.

183 Sim, W., Barnard, R. T., Blaskovich, M., & Ziora, Z. M. (2018). Antimicrobial Silver in Medicinal and Consumer Applications: A Patent Review of the Past Decade (2007-2017). Antibiotics (Basel, Switzerland), 7(4), 93. https://doi.org/10.3390/antibiotics7040093

184 Tuli, H. S., Sandhu, S. S., & Sharma, A. K. (2014). Pharmacological and therapeutic potential of Cordyceps with special reference to Cordycepin. 3 Biotech, 4(1), 1–12. https://doi.org/10.1007/s13205-013-0121-9

185 Chakraborty, A. J., Uddin, T. M., Matin Zidan, B., Mitra, S., Das, R., Nainu, F., Dhama, K., Roy, A., Hossain, M. J., Khusro, A., & Emran, T. B. (2022). Allium cepa: A Treasure of Bioactive Phytochemicals with Prospective Health Benefits. Evidence-based complementary and alternative medicine eCAM, 2022, 4586318. https://doi.org/10.1155/2022/4586318

186 Shingnaisui, K., Dey, T., Manna, P., & Kalita, J. (2018). Therapeutic potentials of Houttuynia cordata Thunb. against inflammation and oxidative stress: A review. Journal of Ethnopharmacology, 220, 35–43. https://doi.org/10.1016/j.jep.2018.03.038

187 Uchide, N., Ohyama, K., Bessho, T., Yuan, B., & Yamakawa, T. (2002). Effect of antioxidants on apoptosis induced by influenza virus infection: inhibition of viral gene replication and transcription with pyrrolidine dithiocarbamate. Antiviral Research, 56(3), 207–217. https://doi.org/10.1016/s0166-3542(02)00109-2

188 Geiler, J., Michaelis, M., Naczk, P., Leutz, A., Langer, K., Doerr, H. W., & Cinatl, J., Jr (2010). N-acetyl-L-cysteine (NAC) inhibits virus replication and expression of pro-inflammatory molecules in A549 cells infected with highly pathogenic H5N1 influenza A virus. Biochemical pharmacology, 79(3), 413–420. https://doi.org/10.1016/j.bcp.2009.08.025

189 Melano, I., Kuo, L. L., Lo, Y. C., Sung, P. W., Tien, N., & Su, W. C. (2021). Effects of Basic Amino Acids and Their Derivatives on SARS-CoV-2 and Influenza-A Virus Infection. Viruses, 13(7), 1301. https://doi.org/10.3390/v13071301

190 Matsue, M., Mori, Y., Nagase, S., Sugiyama, Y., Hirano, R., Ogai, K., Ogura, K., Kurihara, S., & Okamoto, S. (2019). Measuring the Antimicrobial Activity of Lauric Acid against Various Bacteria in Human Gut Microbiota Using a New Method. Cell transplantation, 28(12), 1528–1541. https://doi.org/10.1177/0963689719881366

191 Porter, R. S., & Bode, R. F. (2017). A Review of the Antiviral Properties of Black Elder (Sambucus nigra L.) Products. Phytotherapy research: PTR, 31(4), 533–554. https://doi.org/10.1002/ptr.5782

192 Sun, Z. G., Zhao, T. T., Lu, N., Yang, Y. A., & Zhu, H. L. (2019). Research Progress of Glycyrrhizic Acid on Antiviral Activity. Mini Reviews in Medicinal Chemistry, 19(10), 826–832. https://doi.org/10.2174/1389557519666190119111125

193 Micol, V., Caturla, N., Pérez-Fons, L., Más, V., Pérez, L., & Estepa, A. (2005). The olive leaf extract exhibits antiviral activity against viral haemorrhagic septicaemia rhabdovirus (VHSV). Antiviral Research, 66(2-3), 129–136. https://doi.org/10.1016/j.antiviral.2005.02.005

194 Miraj, S., Rafieian-Kopaei, & Kiani, S. (2017). Melissa officinalis L: A Review Study With an Antioxidant Prospective. Journal of Evidence-Based Complementary & Alternative Medicine, 22(3), 385–394. https://doi.org/10.1177/2156587216663433

195 Arora, R., Chawla, R., Marwah, R., Arora, P., Sharma, R. K., Kaushik, V., Goel, R., Kaur, A., Silambarasan, M., Tripathi, R. P., & Bhardwaj, J. R. (2011). Potential of Complementary and Alternative Medicine in Preventive Management of Novel H1N1 Flu (Swine Flu) Pandemic: Thwarting Potential Disasters in the Bud. Evidence-Based Complementary and Alternative Medicine: eCAM, 2011, 586506. https://doi.org/10.1155/2011/586506

196 Eryılmaz, Met al. (2018). Antimicrobial Activity of Grapefruit Seed. Hacettepe University Journal of the Faculty of Pharmacy. 38. 1-3.

197 Manohar, V., Ingram, C., Gray, J., Talpur, N. A., Echard, B. W., Bagchi, D., & Preuss, H. G. (2001). Antifungal activities of origanum oil against Candida albicans. Molecular and cellular biochemistry, 228(1-2), 111–117. https://doi.org/10.1023/a:1013311632207

198 Hofling, J, et al. (2010). Antimicrobial potential of some plant extracts against Candida species. Braz J Biol. 2010 Nov; 70(4): 1065-8.

199 Vediyappan, G., Dumontet, V., Pelissier, F., & d'Enfert, C. (2013). Gymnemic acids inhibit hyphal growth and virulence in Candida albicans. PloS one, 8(9), e74189. https://doi.org/10.1371/journal.pone.0074189

200 Kumar, S. N., Mani, U. V., & Mani, I. (2010). An open label study on the supplementation of Gymnema sylvestre in type 2 diabetics. Journal of dietary supplements, 7(3), 273–282. https://doi.org/10.3109/19390211.2010.505901

201 Valipe, S. R., Nadeau, J. A., Annamali, T., Venkitanarayanan, K., & Hoagland, T. (2011). In vitro antimicrobial properties of caprylic acid, monocaprylin, and sodium caprylate against Dermatophilus congolensis. American journal of veterinary research, 72(3), 331–335. https://doi.org/10.2460/ajvr.72.3.331

202 Muangphrom, P., Seki, H., Fukushima, E. O., & Muranaka, T. (2016). Artemisinin-based antimalarial research: application of biotechnology to the production of artemisinin, its mode of action, and the mechanism of resistance of Plasmodium parasites. Journal of natural medicines, 70(3), 318–334. https://doi.org/10.1007/s11418-016-1008-y

203 Jahanban-Esfahlan, A., Ostadrahimi, A., Tabibiazar, M., & Amarowicz, R. (2019). A Comprehensive Review on the Chemical Constituents and Functional Uses of Walnut (Juglans spp.) Husk. International journal of molecular sciences, 20(16), 3920. https://doi.org/10.3390/ijms20163920

204 Robinson, R. D., Williams, L. A., Lindo, J. F., Terry, S. I., & Mansingh, A. (1990). Inactivation of strongyloides stercoralis filariform larvae in vitro by six Jamaican plant extracts and three commercial anthelmintics. The West Indian Medical Journal, 39(4), 213–217.

205 Grzybek, M., Kukula-Koch, W., Strachecka, A., Jaworska, A., Phiri, A. M., Paleolog, J., & Tomczuk, K. (2016). Evaluation of Anthelmintic Activity and Composition of Pumpkin (Cucurbita pepo L.) Seed Extracts-In Vitro and in Vivo Studies. International Journal of Molecular Sciences, 17(9), 1456. https://doi.org/10.3390/ijms17091456

Step 2: Immunotherapy

HDCs: Helminth Therapy

206 Parker, W & Ollerton, J. (2013). Evolutionary biology and anthropology suggest biome reconstitution as a necessary approach toward dealing with immune disorders, Evolution, Medicine, and Public Health, 2013, 1; 89–103

207 Turner, W, et al. (2004). Global Urbanization and the Separation of Humans from Nature, BioScience, Volume 54, Issue 6, June 2004, Pages 585–590, https://doi.org/10.1641/0006-3568(2004)054[0585:GUATSO]2.0.CO; 2

208 Van den Elsen, L. W., Garssen, J., Burcelin, R., & Verhasselt, V. (2019). Shaping the gut microbiota by breastfeeding: The gateway to allergy prevention? Frontiers in Pediatrics, 7. https://doi.org/10.3389/fped.2019.00047

209 Biasucci, G., Rubini, M., Riboni, S., Morelli, L., Bessi, E., & Retetangos, C. (2010). Mode of delivery affects the bacterial community in the newborn gut. Early Human Development, 86 Suppl 1, 13–15. https://doi.org/10.1016/j.earlhumdev.2010.01.004

210 Thavagnanam, S, Fleming, J, Bromley, A, Shields, MD, Cardwell, CR. (2008). A meta-analysis of the association between Caesarean section and childhood asthma. Clin Exp Allergy. 2008; 38(4): 629-633.

211 Graham-Rowe, D. Lifestyle: When allergies go west. Nature 479, S2–S4 (2011). https://doi.org/10.1038/479S2a

212 Williamson, et al. (2016). Got worms? Perinatal exposure to helminths prevents persistent immune sensitization and cognitive dysfunction induced by early-life infection. Brain, Behavior and Immunity, January 2016 (51); 14-28

213 Valesquez-Manoff, M. (2012) An epidemic of absence: a new way of understanding allergies and autoimmune diseases. 1st Scribner hardcover ed. New York, NY: Scribner.

214 Bilbo, S. D., Wray, G. A., Perkins, S. E., & Parker, W. (2011). Reconstitution of the human biome as the most reasonable solution for epidemics of allergic and autoimmune diseases. Medical Hypotheses, 77(4), 494–504. https://doi.org/10.1016/j.mehy.2011.06.019

215 Strachan, DP. (1989). Hay fever, hygiene, and household size. BMJ. 1989; 299(6710): 1259-1260.

216 Abdoli, A., & Mirzaian Ardakani, H. (2020). Potential application of helminth therapy for resolution of neuroinflammation in neuropsychiatric disorders. Metabolic Brain Disease, 35(1), 95–110. https://doi.org/10.1007/s11011-019-00466-5

217 Kelly, J. R., Minuto, C., Cryan, J. F., Clarke, G., & Dinan, T. G. (2017). Cross Talk: The Microbiota and Neurodevelopmental Disorders. Frontiers in Neuroscience, 11, 490. https://doi.org/10.3389/fnins.2017.00490

218 Shi, W., Xu, N., Wang, X., Vallée, I., Liu, M., & Liu, X. (2022). Helminth Therapy for Immune-Mediated Inflammatory Diseases: Current and Future Perspectives. Journal of inflammation research, 15, 475–491. https://doi.org/10.2147/JIR.S348079

219 Maizels, RM, McSorley, HJ. (2016). Regulation of the host immune system by helminth parasites. The Journal of Allergy and Clinical Immunology. 2016; 138(3): 666-675. doi:10.1016/j.jaci.2016.07.007.

220 Smallwood, T. B., Giacomin, P. R., Loukas, A., Mulvenna, J. P., Clark, R. J., & Miles, J. J. (2017). Helminth Immunomodulation in Autoimmune Disease. Frontiers in Immunology, 8, 453. https://doi.org/10.3389/fimmu.2017.00453

Inflammation

221 Pérez-Vigil, A., Fernández de la Cruz, L., Brander, G., Isomura, K., Gromark, C., & Mataix-Cols, D. (2016). The link between autoimmune diseases and obsessive-compulsive and tic disorders: A systematic review. Neuroscience and biobehavioral reviews, 71, 542–562. https://doi.org/10.1016/j.neubiorev.2016.09.025

222 Kiessling, L. S., Marcotte, A. C., & Culpepper, L. (1993). Antineuronal antibodies in movement disorders. Pediatrics, 92(1), 39–43.

223 Kirvan, C. A., Swedo, S. E., Heuser, J. S., & Cunningham, M. W. (2003). Mimicry and autoantibody-mediated neuronal cell signaling in Sydenham chorea. Nature medicine, 9(7), 914–920. https://doi.org/10.1038/nm892

224 Church, A. J., Dale, R. C., & Giovannoni, G. (2004). Anti-basal ganglia antibodies: a possible diagnostic utility in idiopathic movement disorders? Archives of Disease in Childhood, 89(7), 611–614. https://doi.org/10.1136/adc.2003.031880

225 Chang, K., Frankovich, J., Cooperstock, M., Cunningham, M. W., Latimer, M. E., Murphy, T. K., Pasternack, M., Thienemann, M., Williams, K., Walter, J., Swedo, S. E., & PANS Collaborative Consortium (2015). Clinical evaluation of youth with pediatric acute-onset neuropsychiatric syndrome (PANS): recommendations from the 2013 PANS Consensus Conference. Journal of Child and Adolescent Psychopharmacology, 25(1), 3–13. https://doi.org/10.1089/cap.2014.0084

226 Cox, C. J., Zuccolo, A. J., Edwards, E. V., Mascaro-Blanco, A., Alvarez, K., Stoner, J., Chang, K., & Cunningham, M. W. (2015). Antineuronal antibodies in a heterogeneous group of youth and young adults with tics and obsessive-compulsive disorder. Journal of Child and Adolescent Psychopharmacology, 25(1), 76–85. https://doi.org/10.1089/cap.2014.0048

227 Chain, J, et al. (2020). Autoantibody Biomarkers for Basal Ganglia Encephalitis in Sydenham Chorea and Pediatric Autoimmune Neuropsychiatric Disorder Associated With Streptococcal Infections. Frontiers in Psychiatry. Vol 11 https://doi.org/10.3389/fpsyt.2020.00564

228 Ravin, K. A., & Loy, M. (2015). The Eosinophil in Infection. Clinical Reviews in Allergy & Immunology, 50(2), 214–227. https://doi.org/10.1007/s12016-015-8525-4

229 Shea-Donohue, T., Stiltz, J., Zhao, A., & Notari, L. (2010). Mast cells. Current gastroenterology reports, 12(5), 349–357. https://doi.org/10.1007/s11894-010-0132-1

230 Malone, R. W., Tisdall, P., Fremont-Smith, P., Liu, Y., Huang, X. P., White, K. M., Miorin, L., Moreno, E., Alon, A., Delaforge, E., Hennecker, C. D., Wang, G., Pottel, J., Blair, R. V., Roy, C. J., Smith, N., Hall, J. M., Tomera, K. M., Shapiro,

G., Mittermaier, A., ... Ricke, D. O. (2021). COVID-19: Famotidine, Histamine, Mast Cells, and Mechanisms. Frontiers in Pharmacology, 12, 633680. https://doi.org/10.3389/fphar.2021.633680

231 Castells, M., & Austen, K. F. (2002). Mastocytosis: mediator-related signs and symptoms. International Archives of Allergy and Immunology, 127(2), 147–152. https://doi.org/10.1159/000048188

232 Theoharides, T. C., Tsilioni, I., & Ren, H. (2019). Recent advances in our understanding of mast cell activation or should it be mast cell mediator disorders?. Expert Review of Clinical Immunology, 15(6), 639–656. https://doi.org/10.1080/1744666X.2019.1596800

233 Babu, K. S., Polosa, R., & Morjaria, J. B. (2013). Anti-IgE--emerging opportunities for Omalizumab. Expert Opinion on Biological Therapy, 13(5), 765–777. https://doi.org/10.1517/14712598.2013.782391

234 Xu, J., Liu, R. J., Fahey, S., Frick, L., Leckman, J., Vaccarino, F., Duman, R. S., Williams, K., Swedo, S., & Pittenger, C. (2021). Antibodies From Children With PANDAS Bind Specifically to Striatal Cholinergic Interneurons and Alter Their Activity. The American Journal of Psychiatry, 178(1), 48–64. https://doi.org/10.1176/appi.ajp.2020.19070698

235 Frick, L., & Pittenger, C. (2016). Microglial Dysregulation in OCD, Tourette Syndrome, and PANDAS. Journal of Immunology Research, 8606057. https://doi.org/10.1155/2016/8606057

236 Sears, B. (2015). Anti-inflammatory Diets. Journal of the American College of Nutrition, 34 Suppl 1, 14–21. https://doi.org/10.1080/07315724.2015.1080105

237 Theophilus, P. A., Victoria, M. J., Socarras, K. M., Filush, K. R., Gupta, K., Luecke, D. F., & Sapi, E. (2015). Effectiveness of Stevia Rebaudiana Whole Leaf Extract Against the Various Morphological Forms of Borrelia Burgdorferi in Vitro. European Journal of Microbiology & Immunology, 5(4), 268–280. https://doi.org/10.1556/1886.2015.00031

238 Gaweł-Bęben, K., Bujak, T., Nizioł-Łukaszewska, Z., Antosiewicz, B., Jakubczyk, A., Karaś, M., & Rybczyńska, K. (2015). Stevia rebaudiana Bert. leaf extracts as a multifunctional source of natural antioxidants. Molecules (Basel, Switzerland), 20(4), 5468–5486. https://doi.org/10.3390/molecules20045468

239 Vernino, S, et al. (2021). Postural orthostatic tachycardia syndrome (POTS): State of the science and clinical care from a 2019 National Institutes of Health Expert Consensus Meeting Part 1, Autonomic Neuroscience, Volume 235, 102828, ISSN 1566-0702, https://doi.org/10.1016/j.autneu.2021.102828.

240 Raj, S.R., et al. (2021). Postural orthostatic tachycardia syndrome (POTS): Priorities for POTS care and research from a 2019 National Institutes of Health Expert Consensus Meeting Part 2 Autonomic Neuroscience: Basic and Clinical, Volume 235

241 Maroon, JC & Bost, J. (2006). Fish Oil: the Natural Anti-Inflammatory. Laguna Beach, CA: Basic Health Publications

242 Yang, A., Wu, Y., Yu, G., & Wang, H. (2021). Role of specialized pro-resolving lipid mediators in pulmonary inflammation diseases: mechanisms and development. Respiratory Research, 22(1), 204. https://doi.org/10.1186/s12931-021-01792-y

243 Langmead, L., Makins, R. J., & Rampton, D. S. (2004). Anti-inflammatory effects of aloe vera gel in human colorectal mucosa in vitro. Alimentary Pharmacology & Therapeutics, 19(5), 521–527. https://doi.org/10.1111/j.1365-2036.2004.01874.x

244 Lopresti, AL, Maes, M, Maker, GL, Hood, SD & Drummond, PD. (2014). Curcumin for the treatment of major depression: a randomised, double-blind, placebo controlled study. J Affect Disord; 167:368-375. doi:10.1016/j.jad.2014.06.001

245 Panche, A. N., Diwan, A. D., & Chandra, S. R. (2016). Flavonoids: an overview. Journal of Nutritional Science, 5, e47. https://doi.org/10.1017/jns.2016.41

246 Pryimak, N., Zaiachuk, M., Kovalchuk, O., & Kovalchuk, I. (2021). The Potential Use of Cannabis in Tissue Fibrosis. Frontiers in Cell and Developmental Biology, 9, 715380. https://doi.org/10.3389/fcell.2021.715380

247 Belluzzi, A, Brignola, C, Campieri, M, et al.(1994). Effects of new fish oil derivative on fatty acid phospholipid-membrane pattern in a group of Crohn's disease patients. Dig Dis Sci; 39(12): 2589-2594. doi:10.1007/BF02087694

248 Calder, PC. (2010). Omega-3 fatty acids and inflammatory processes. Nutrients; 2(3): 355-374. doi:10.3390/nu2030355

249 Chang, C. Y., Ke, D. S., & Chen, J. Y. (2009). Essential fatty acids and human brain. Acta neurologica Taiwanica, 18(4), 231–241.

250 Huss, M, Völp, A, Stauss-Grabo, M. (2010). Supplementation of polyunsaturated fatty acids, magnesium and zinc in children seeking medical advice for attention-deficit/hyperactivity problems an observational cohort study. Lipids Health Dis. 2010;9:105. Published 2010 Sep 24. doi:10.1186/1476-511X-9-105

251 Shang, P., Zhang, Y., Ma, D., Hao, Y., Wang, X., Xin, M., Zhang, Y., Zhu, M., & Feng, J. (2019). Inflammation resolution and specialized pro-resolving lipid mediators in CNS diseases. Expert opinion on therapeutic targets, 23(11), 967–986. https://doi.org/10.1080/14728222.2019.1691525

252 Naini, M. A., Zargari-Samadnejad, A., Mehrvarz, S., Tanideh, R., Ghorbani, M., Dehghanian, A., Hasanzarrini, M., Banaee, F., Koohi-Hosseinabadi, O., Tanideh, N., & Iraji, A. (2021). Anti-Inflammatory, Antioxidant, and Healing-Promoting Effects of Aloe vera Extract in the Experimental Colitis in Rats. Evidence-based complementary and alternative medicine eCAM, 2021, 9945244. https://doi.org/10.1155/2021/9945244

253 Guo, X., & Mei, N. (2016). Aloe vera: A review of toxicity and adverse clinical effects. Journal of Environmental Science and Health. Part C, Environmental carcinogenesis & ecotoxicology reviews, 34(2), 77–96. https://doi.org/10.1080/10590501.2016.1166826

254 Daily, J. W., Yang, M., & Park, S. (2016). Efficacy of Turmeric Extracts and Curcumin for Alleviating the Symptoms of Joint Arthritis: A Systematic Review and Meta-Analysis of Randomized Clinical Trials. Journal of Medicinal Food, 19(8), 717–729. https://doi.org/10.1089/jmf.2016.3705

255 Sunagawa, Y., Hirano, S., Katanasaka, Y., Miyazaki, Y., Funamoto, M., Okamura, N., Hojo, Y., Suzuki, H., Doi, O., Yokoji, T., Morimoto, E., Takashi, T., Ozawa, H., Imaizumi, A., Ueno, M., Kakeya, H., Shimatsu, A., Wada, H., Hasegawa, K., & Morimoto, T. (2015). Colloidal submicron-particle curcumin exhibits high absorption efficiency-a double-blind, 3-way crossover study. Journal of Nutritional Science and Vitaminology, 61(1), 37–44. https://doi.org/10.3177/jnsv.61.37

256 Panahi, Y., Kianpour, P., Mohtashami, R., Jafari, R., Simental-Mendía, L. E., & Sahebkar, A. (2017). Efficacy and Safety of Phytosomal Curcumin in Non-Alcoholic Fatty Liver Disease: A Randomized Controlled Trial. Drug research, 67(4), 244–251. https://doi.org/10.1055/s-0043-100019

257 Bhawana, Basniwal, R. K., Buttar, H. S., Jain, V. K., & Jain, N. (2011). Curcumin nanoparticles: preparation, characterization, and antimicrobial study. Journal of Agricultural and Food Chemistry, 59(5), 2056–2061. https://doi.org/10.1021/jf104402t

258 Di Meo, F., Filosa, S., Madonna, M., Giello, G., Di Pardo, A., Maglione, V., Baldi, A., & Crispi, S. (2019). Curcumin C3 complex®/Bioperine® has antineoplastic activity in mesothelioma: an in vitro and in vivo analysis. Journal of Experimental & Clinical Cancer Research CR, 38(1), 360. https://doi.org/10.1186/s13046-019-1368-8

259 Theoharides, T. C., Asadi, S., & Panagiotidou, S. (2012). A case series of a luteolin formulation (NeuroProtek®) in children with autism spectrum disorders. International Journal of Immunopathology and Pharmacology, 25(2), 317–323. https://doi.org/10.1177/039463201202500201

260 Maleki, S. J., Crespo, J. F., & Cabanillas, B. (2019). Anti-inflammatory effects of flavonoids. Food Chemistry, 299, 125124. https://doi.org/10.1016/j.foodchem.2019.125124

261 Atalay, S., Jarocka-Karpowicz, I., & Skrzydlewska, E. (2019). Antioxidative and Anti-Inflammatory Properties of Cannabidiol. Antioxidants (Basel, Switzerland), 9(1), 21. https://doi.org/10.3390/antiox9010021

262 Casarotto, PC, Gomes, FV, Resstel, LB, Guimarães, FS. (2010). Cannabidiol inhibitory effect on marble-burying behaviour: involvement of CB1 receptors. Behav Pharmacol. 2010; 21(4): 353-358. doi:10.1097/fbp.0b013e32833b33c5

263 Zieba J, Sinclair D, Sebree T, et al. (2019). Cannabidiol (CBD) reduces anxiety-related behavior in mice via an FMRP-independent mechanism. Pharmacol Biochem Behav. 2019; 181: 93-100. doi:10.1016/j.pbb.2019.05.002

264 Chincholkar M. (2018). Analgesic mechanisms of gabapentinoids and effects in experimental pain models: a narrative review. British Journal of Anaesthesia. Vol 120 (6): 1315-1334. doi: 10.1016/j.bja.2018.02.066

265 Berlin, R. K., Butler, P. M., & Perloff, M. D. (2015). Gabapentin Therapy in Psychiatric Disorders: A Systematic Review. The Primary Care Companion for CNS Disorders, 17(5), 10.4088/PCC.15r01821. https://doi.org/10.4088/PCC.15r01821

266 Markota, M., & Morgan, R. J. (2017). Treatment of Generalized Anxiety Disorder with Gabapentin. Case Reports in Psychiatry, 2017, 6045017. https://doi.org/10.1155/2017/6045017

267 Peckham, A. M., Evoy, K. E., Ochs, L., & Covvey, J. R. (2018). Gabapentin for Off-Label Use: Evidence-Based or Cause for Concern?. Substance Abuse: Research and Treatment, 12, 1178221818801311. https://doi.org/10.1177/1178221818801311

268 Frankovich, J., Swedo, S., Murphy, T., Dale, R. C., Agalliu, D., Williams, K., Daines, M., Hornig, M., Chugani, H., Sanger, T., Muscal, E., Pasternack, M., Cooperstock, M., Gans, H., Zhang, Y., Cunningham, M., Bernstein, G., Bromberg, R., Willett, T., Thienemann, M. (2017). Clinical management of pediatric acute-onset neuropsychiatric syndrome: Part II—use of immunomodulatory therapies. Journal of Child and Adolescent Psychopharmacology, 27(7), 574-593. https://doi.org/10.1089/cap.2016.0148

269 Shin, Y. W., Lee, S. T., Park, K. I., Jung, K. H., Jung, K. Y., Lee, S. K., & Chu, K. (2017). Treatment strategies for autoimmune encephalitis. Therapeutic Advances in Neurological Disorders, 11, 1756285617722347. https://doi.org/10.1177/1756285617722347

270 Kovacevic, M., Grant, P., & Swedo, S. E. (2015). Use of intravenous immunoglobulin in the treatment of twelve youths with pediatric autoimmune neuropsychiatric disorders associated with Streptococcal infections. Journal of Child and Adolescent Psychopharmacology, 25(1), 65–69. https://doi.org/10.1089/cap.2014.0067

271 Garvey, M. A., Snider, L. A., Leitman, S. F., Werden, R., & Swedo, S. E. (2005). Treatment of Sydenham's chorea with intravenous immunoglobulin, plasma exchange, or prednisone. Journal of Child Neurology, 20(5), 424–429. https://doi.org/10.1177/08830738050200050601

272 Latimer, M. E., L'Etoile, N., Seidlitz, J., & Swedo, S. E. (2015). Therapeutic Plasma Apheresis as A Treatment For 35 Severely Ill Children and Adolescents With Pediatric Autoimmune Neuropsychiatric Disorders Associated With Streptococcal Infections. Journal of Child and Adolescent Psychopharmacology, 25(1), 70–75.https://doi.org/10.1089/cap.2014.0080

273 Frankovich, J., Swedo, S. E., Murphy, T., Dale, R. C., Agalliu, D., Williams, K., Daines, M., Hornig, M., Chugani, H., Sanger, T., Muscal, E., Pasternack, M., Cooperstock, M., Gans, H., Zhang, Y., Cunningham, M., Bernstein, G., Bromberg, R., Willett, T., Brown, K., Farhadian, B., Chang, K., Geller, D., Hernandez, J., Sherr, J., Shaw, R., Latimer, E., Leckman, J., Thienemann, M., & PANS/PANDAS Consortium (2017). Clinical Management of Pediatric AcuteOnset Neuropsychiatric Syndrome: Part II-Use of Immunomodulatory Therapies. Journal of Child and Adolescent Psychopharmacology, 27(7), 574-593. https://doi.org/10.1089/cap.2016.0148.

274 Walker, A. R., Tani, L. Y., Thompson, J. A., Firth, S. D., Veasy, L. G., & Bale, J. F., Jr (2007). Rheumatic chorea: relationship to systemic manifestations and response to corticosteroids. The Journal of Pediatrics, 151(6), 679–683. https://doi.org/10.1016/j.jpeds.2007.04.059

275 Chadeganipour, M., & Mohammadi, R. (2015). Steroid-binding receptors in fungi: implication for systemic mycoses. Current Medical Mycology, 1(2), 46–52. https://doi.org/10.18869/acadpub.cmm.1.2.46

276 Perlmutter, S. J., Leitman, S. F., Garvey, M. A., Hamburger, S., Feldman, E., Leonard, H. L., & Swedo, S. E. (1999). Therapeutic plasma exchange and intravenous immunoglobulin for obsessive-compulsive disorder and tic disorders in childhood. Lancet (London, England), 354(9185), 1153–1158. https://doi.org/10.1016/S0140-6736(98)12297-3

277 Melamed, I, et al. (2021). Evaluation of Intravenous Immunoglobulin in Pediatric Acute-Onset Neuropsychiatric Syndrome. Journal of Child and Adolescent Psychopharmacology. Mar 2021.118-128.http://doi.org/10.1089/cap.2020.0100

278 Pavone, P., Falsaperla, R., Nicita, F., Zecchini, A., Battaglia, C., Spalice, A., Iozzi, L., Parano, E., Vitaliti, G., Verrotti, A., Belcastro, V., Cho, S.Y., Jin, D., & Savasta, S. (2018). Pediatric Autoimmune Neuropsychiatric Disorder Associated with Streptococcal Infection (PANDAS): Clinical Manifestations, IVIG Treatment Outcomes, Results from a Cohort of Italian Patients. Neuropsychiatry (London) (2018) 8(1), 739–744

279 Williams, K. A., Swedo, S. E., Farmer, C. A., Grantz, H., Grant, P. J., D'Souza, P., Hommer, R., Katsovich, L., King, R. A., & Leckman, J. F. (2016). Randomized, Controlled Trial of Intravenous Immunoglobulin for Pediatric Autoimmune Neuropsychiatric Disorders Associated With Streptococcal Infections. Journal of the American Academy of Child and Adolescent Psychiatry, 55(10), 860–867.e2. https://doi.org/10.1016/j.jaac.2016.06.017.

280 Vitaliti, G., Tabatabaie, O., Matin, N., Ledda, C., Pavone, P., Lubrano, R., Serra, A., Di Mauro, P., Cocuzza, S., & Falsaperla, R. (2015). The usefulness of immunotherapy in pediatric neurodegenerative disorders: A systematic review of literature data. Human Vaccines & Immunotherapeutics, 11(12), 2749–2763. https://doi.org/10.1080/21645515.2015.1061161

281 Krouse, A, et al. (2021). Plasmapheresis, Rituximab, and Ceftriaxone Provided Lasting Improvement for a 27-Year-Old Adult Male with Pediatric Autoimmune Neuropsychiatric Disorders Associated with Streptococcal Infections (PANDAS). Case Reports in Psychiatry, vol. 2021, Article ID 8697902, 4 pages, 2021. https://doi.org/10.1155/2021/8697902

282 Cooperstock, MS, Swedo, SE, Pasternack, MS, et al. (2017). Clinical management of pediatric acute-onset neuropsychiatric syndrome: part III-treatment and prevention of infections. J Child Adol Psychop. 2017; 27: 594–606

283 Endres, D., Pollak, T.A., Bechter, K. et al. (2022). Immunological causes of obsessive-compulsive disorder: is it time for the concept of an "autoimmune OCD" subtype?.Transl Psychiatry 12, 5. https://doi.org/10.1038/s41398-021-01700-4

The Addition of Antioxidants

284 Lee, K. H., Cha, M., & Lee, B. H. (2020). Neuroprotective Effect of Antioxidants in the Brain. International Journal of Molecular Sciences, 21(19), 7152. https://doi.org/10.3390/ijms21197152

285 Arulselvan, P., Fard, M. T., Tan, W. S., Gothai, S., Fakurazi, S., Norhaizan, M. E., & Kumar, S. S. (2016). Role of Antioxidants and Natural Products in Inflammation. Oxidative Medicine and Cellular Longevity; 5276130. https://doi.org/10.1155/2016/5276130

286 Fiedor, J., & Burda, K. (2014). Potential role of carotenoids as antioxidants in human health and disease. Nutrients, 6(2), 466–488. https://doi.org/10.3390/nu6020466

287 Stephensen C. B. (2001). Vitamin A, infection, and immune function. Annual Review of Nutrition, 21, 167–192. https://doi.org/10.1146/annurev.nutr.21.1.167

288 Lee, H., & Ko, G. (2017). New perspectives regarding the antiviral effect of vitamin A on norovirus using modulation of gut microbiota. Gut Microbes, 8(6), 616–620. https://doi.org/10.1080/19490976.2017.1353842

289 Sommer, A. (2008). Vitamin A Deficiency and Clinical Disease: An Historical Overview, The Journal of Nutrition, Volume 138, Issue 10, October 2008, Pages 1835–1839, https://doi.org/10.1093/jn/138.10.1835

290 McCandless, J., Binstock, T., & Zimmerman, J. (2003). Children with starving brains: A medical treatment guide for autism spectrum disorder. Bramble Company.

291 Carr, A. C., & Maggini, S. (2017). Vitamin C and Immune Function. Nutrients, 9(11), 1211. https://doi.org/10.3390/nu9111211

292 Hemilä, H. (2017). Vitamin C and Infections. Nutrients. 2017; 9(4): 339. Published 2017 Mar 29. doi:10.3390/nu9040339

293 Kumar, A., R. V. Saini, and A. K. Saini. (2018). Neuroprotective Role of Ascorbic Acid: Antioxidant and Non-antioxidant Functions. Asian Journal of Pharmaceutical and Clinical Research, Vol. 11, no. 10, Oct. 2018, pp. 30-33, doi:10.22159/ajpcr.2018.v11i10.27318

294 Martineau, A. R., Jolliffe, D. A., Hooper, R. L., Greenberg, L., Aloia, J. F., Bergman, P., Dubnov-Raz, G., Esposito, S., Ganmaa, D., Ginde, A. A., Goodall, E. C., Grant, C. C., Griffiths, C. J., Janssens, W., Laaksi, I., Manaseki-Holland, S., Mauger, D., Murdoch, D. R., Neale, R., Rees, J. R., … Camargo, C. A., Jr (2017). Vitamin D supplementation to prevent acute respiratory tract infections: systematic review and meta-analysis of individual participant data. BMJ (Clinical research ed.), 356, i6583. https://doi.org/10.1136/bmj.i6583

295 Hewison, M. (2012). Vitamin D and immune function: an overview. The Proceedings of the Nutrition Society, 71(1), 50–61. https://doi.org/10.1017/S0029665111001650

296 Esposito, S., & Lelii, M. (2015). Vitamin D and respiratory tract infections in childhood. BMC Infectious Diseases, 15, 487. https://doi.org/10.1186/s12879-015-1196-1

297 Lopez-Munoz, P, Beltran, B, Saez-Gonzalez, E, Alba, A, Nos, P, Iborra, M. (2019). Influence of vitamin D deficiency on inflammatory markers and clinical disease activity in IBD patients. Nutrients. 2019; 11: 1059. doi: 10.3390/nu11051059

298 Stagi, S, Lepri, G, Rigante, D, Matucci Cerinic, M, & Falcini, F. (2018). Cross-Sectional Evaluation of Plasma Vitamin D Levels in a Large Cohort of Italian Patients with Pediatric Autoimmune Neuropsychiatric Disorders Associated with Streptococcal Infections. Journal of Child and Adolescent Psychopharmacology, 28(2), 124–129. https://doi.org/10.1089/cap.2016.0159

299 Charoenngam, N, & Holick, MF. (2020). Immunologic Effects of Vitamin D on Human Health and Disease. Nutrients, 12(7), 2097. https://doi.org/10.3390/nu12072097

300 Holmøy, T & Moen, SM. (2010). Assessing vitamin D in the central nervous system. Acta neurologica Scandinavica. Supplementum, (190), 88–92. https://doi.org/10.1111/j.1600-0404.2010.01383.x

301 Berridge, MJ. (2015). Vitamin D cell signalling in health and disease. Biochemical and biophysical research communications, 460(1), 53–71. https://doi.org/10.1016/j.bbrc.2015.01.008

302 Jain, SK, & Micinski, D. (2013). Vitamin D upregulates glutamate cysteine ligase and glutathione reductase, and GSH formation, and decreases ROS and MCP-1 and IL-8 secretion in high-glucose exposed U937 monocytes. Biochemical and Biophysical Research Communications, 437(1), 7–11. https://doi.org/10.1016/j.bbrc.2013.06.004

303 Velthuis, AJ, van den Worm, SH, Sims, AC, Baric, RS, Snijder, EJ, & van Hemert, MJ. (2010). Zn(2+) inhibits coronavirus and arterivirus RNA polymerase activity in vitro and zinc ionophores block the replication of these viruses in cell culture. PLoS pathogens, 6(11), e1001176. https://doi.org/10.1371/journal.ppat.1001176

304 Maares, M, & Haase, H. (2016). Zinc and immunity: An essential interrelation. Archives of Biochemistry and Biophysics, 611, 58–65. https://doi.org/10.1016/j.abb.2016.03.022

305 Prasad AS. (2014). Impact of the discovery of human zinc deficiency on health. Journal of Trace Elements in Medicine and Biology: organ of the Society for Minerals and Trace Elements (GMS), 28(4), 357–363. https://doi.org/10.1016/j.jtemb.2014.09.002

306 Wang, L, & Song, Y. (2018). Efficacy of zinc given as an adjunct to the treatment of severe pneumonia: A meta-analysis of randomized, double-blind and placebo-controlled trials. The Clinical Respiratory Journal, 12(3), 857–864. https://doi.org/10.1111/crj.12646

307 Li, DD, Zhang, W, Wang, ZY, & Zhao, P. (2017). Serum Copper, Zinc, and Iron Levels in Patients with Alzheimer's Disease: A Meta-Analysis of Case-Control Studies. Frontiers in Aging Neuroscience, 9, 300. https://doi.org/10.3389/fnagi.2017.00300

308 Huss, M, Völp, A, Stauss-Grabo, M. (2010) Supplementation of polyunsaturated fatty acids, magnesium and zinc in children seeking medical advice for attention-deficit/hyperactivity problems an observational cohort study. Lipids Health Dis. 2010;9:105. Published 2010 Sep 24. doi:10.1186/1476-511X-9-105

309 Mahmoud, MM, El-Mazary, AA, Maher, RM, Saber, MM. (2011) Zinc, ferritin, magnesium and copper in a group of Egyptian children with attention deficit hyperactivity disorder. Ital J Pediatr. 2011; 37: 60. Published 2011 Dec 29. doi:10.1186/1824-7288-37-60

310 Oner, O, Oner, P, Bozkurt, OH, et al. (2010) Effects of zinc and ferritin levels on parent and teacher reported symptom scores in attention deficit hyperactivity disorder. Child Psychiatry Hum Dev. 2010; 41(4): 441-447. doi:10.1007/s10578-010-0178-1

311 Lin, SC, Ho, C.T, Chuo, WH, Li, S, Wang, T T, & Lin, CC. (2017). Effective inhibition of MERS-CoV infection by resveratrol. BMC Infectious Diseases, 17(1), 144. https://doi.org/10.1186/s12879-017-2253-8

312 Ramdani, LH, & Bachari, K. (2020). Potential therapeutic effects of Resveratrol against SARS-CoV-2. Acta virologica, 64(3), 276–280. https://doi.org/10.4149/av_2020_309

313 Vestergaard, M, & Ingmer, H. (2019). Antibacterial and antifungal properties of resveratrol. International Journal of Antimicrobial Agents, 53(6), 716–723. https://doi.org/10.1016/j.ijantimicag.2019.02.015

314 Tordjman, S, Chokron, S, Delorme, R, Charrier, A, Bellissant, E, Jaafari, N & Fougerou, C. (2017). Melatonin: Pharmacology, Functions and Therapeutic Benefits. Current Neuropharmacology, 15(3), 434–443. https://doi.org/10.2174/1570159X14666161228122115

315 Reiter, R J, Mayo, JC, Tan, DX,, Sainz, RM, Alatorre-Jimenez, M, & Qin, L. (2016). Melatonin as an antioxidant: under promises but over delivers. Journal of Pineal Research, 61(3), 253–278. https://doi.org/10.1111/jpi.12360

316 Gurunathan, S, Kang, MH., Choi, Y, Reiter, RJ & Kim, JH. (2021). Melatonin: A potential therapeutic agent against COVID-19. Melatonin Research. 4, 1 (Jan. 2021), 30-69. DOI:https://doi.org/https://doi.org/10.32794/mr11250081.

317 Pizzorno J. (2014). Glutathione!. Integrative Medicine (Encinitas, Calif.), 13(1), 8–12.

318 James, SJ, Melnyk, S, Jernigan, S, Hubanks, A, Rose, S, Gaylor, DW. (2008). Abnormal transmethylation/transsulfuration metabolism and DNA hypomethylation among parents of children with autism. J Autism Dev Disord. 2008 Nov; 38(10): 1966-75. doi: 10.1007/s10803-008-0591-5

319 James, SJ, Cutler, P, Melnyk, S, Jernigan, S, Janak, L, Gaylor, DW & Neubrander, JA. (2004). Metabolic biomarkers of increased oxidative stress and impaired methylation capacity in children with autism. The American Journal of Clinical Nutrition, 80(6), 1611–1617. https://doi.org/10.1093/ajcn/80.6.1611

320 Ajmone-Cat, MA, Spinello, C, Valenti, D, Franchi, F, Macrì, S, Vacca, RA, Laviola, G. (2019). Brain-Immune Alterations and Mitochondrial Dysfunctions in a Mouse Model of Paediatric Autoimmune Disorder Associated with Streptococcus: Exacerbation by Chronic Psychosocial Stress. Journal of Clinical Medicine; 8(10): 1514. https://doi.org/10.3390/jcm8101514

321 Murgia, F, et al. (2021). Metabolomic Characterization of Pediatric Acute-Onset Neuropsychiatric Syndrome (PANS). Frontiers in Neuroscience. Vol 15. DOI: 10.3389/fnins.2021.645267

322 Lauterburg, BH. (2002). Analgesics and glutathione. American Journal of Therapeutics, 9(3), 225–233. https://doi.org/10.1097/00045391-200205000-00008

323 Richie, JP, Jr, Nichenametla, S, Neidig, W, Calcagnotto, A, Haley, JS, Schell, TD & Muscat, JE. (2015). Randomized controlled trial of oral glutathione supplementation on body stores of glutathione. European Journal of Nutrition, 54(2), 251–263. https://doi.org/10.1007/s00394-014-0706-z

324 Benzie, IF & Choi, SW. (2014). Antioxidants in food: content, measurement, significance, action, cautions, caveats, and research needs. Advances in Food and Nutrition Research, 71, 1–53. https://doi.org/10.1016/B978-0-12-800270-4.00001-8

325 Wilson, DW, Nash, P, Buttar, HS, Griffiths, K, Singh, R, De Meester, F, Horiuchi, R & Takahashi, T. (2017). The Role of Food Antioxidants, Benefits of Functional Foods, and Influence of Feeding Habits on the Health of the Older Person: An Overview. Antioxidants (Basel, Switzerland), 6(4), 81. https://doi.org/10.3390/antiox6040081

Nutrition

326 Xu, et al. (2019). The Dynamic Interplay between the Gut Microbiota and Autoimmune Disease. Journal of Immunology Research, Oct, 2019.

327 Sonnenburg, E, Smits, S, Tikhonov, M. et al. (2016). Diet-induced extinctions in the gut microbiota compound over generations. Nature 529, 212–215.

328 Penders, J, Gerhold, K, Thijs, C, et al. (2014). New insights into the hygiene hypothesis in allergic diseases: mediation of sibling and birth mode effects by the gut microbiota. Gut Microbes; 5(2): 239-244.

329 Korpela, K, Salonen, A, Virta, L, et al. (2016). Intestinal microbiome is related to lifetime antibiotic use in Finnish preschool children. Nat Commun 7, 10410.

330 Charbonneau, MR, O'Donnell, D, Blanton, LV, et al. (2016). Sialylated Milk Oligosaccharides Promote Microbiota-Dependent Growth in Models of Infant Undernutrition. Cell; 164(5): 859-871.

331 Ayati, Z, Sarris, J, Chang, D, Emami, SA & Rahimi, R. (2020). Herbal medicines and phytochemicals for obsessive-compulsive disorder. Phytotherapy Research PTR, 34(8), 1889–1901. https://doi.org/10.1002/ptr.6656

332 Khodadadegan, MA, Azami, S, Guest, PC, Jamialahmadi, T & Sahebkar, A. (2021). Effects of Curcumin on Depression and Anxiety: A Narrative Review of the Recent Clinical Data. Advances in Experimental Medicine and Biology, 1291, 283–294. https://doi.org/10.1007/978-3-030-56153-6_17

333 Grzanna, R, Lindmark, L & Frondoza, CG. (2005). Ginger--an herbal medicinal product with broad anti-inflammatory actions. Journal of Medicinal Food, 8(2), 125–132. https://doi.org/10.1089/jmf.2005.8.125

334 Arreola, R, Quintero-Fabián, S, López-Roa, RI, Flores-Gutiérrez, EO, Reyes-Grajeda, JP, Carrera-Quintanar, L & Ortuño-Sahagún, D. (2015). Immunomodulation and anti-inflammatory effects of garlic compounds. Journal of Immunology Research, 2015, 401630. https://doi.org/10.1155/2015/401630

335 Schink, A., Naumoska, K., Kitanovski, Z., Kampf, C. J., Fröhlich-Nowoisky, J., Thines, E., Pöschl, U., Schuppan, D., & Lucas, K., (2018). Anti-inflammatory effects of cinnamon extract and identification of active compounds influencing the TLR2 and TLR4 signaling pathways. Food & function, 9(11), 5950–5964. https://doi.org/10.1039/c8fo01286e

336 Slighoua, M, Mahdi, I, Amrati, FE, Di Cristo, F, Amaghnouje, A, Grafov, A, Boucetta, N, Bari, A, & Bousta, D. (2021). Assessment of in vivo estrogenic and anti-inflammatory activities of the hydro-ethanolic extract and polyphenolic fraction of parsley (Petroselinum sativum Hoffm.). Journal of Ethnopharmacology, 265, 113290. https://doi.org/10.1016/j.jep.2020.113290

337 Rodriguez-Garcia, I, Silva-Espinoza, BA, Ortega-Ramirez, LA, Leyva, JM, Siddiqui, MW, Cruz-Valenzuela, MR, Gonzalez-Aguilar, GA & Ayala-Zavala, JF. (2016). Oregano Essential Oil as an Antimicrobial and Antioxidant Additive in Food Products. Critical Reviews in Food Science and Nutrition, 56(10), 1717–1727. https://doi.org/10.1080/10408398.2013.800832

338 Borugă, O, Jianu, C, Mişcă, C, Goleţ, Gruia, AT & Horhat, FG. (2014). Thymus vulgaris essential oil: chemical composition and antimicrobial activity. Journal of Medicine and Life, 7 Spec No. 3(Spec Iss 3), 56–60.

339 Vasconcelos, NG, Croda, J & Simionatto, S. (2018). Antibacterial mechanisms of cinnamon and its constituents: A review. Microbial Pathogenesis, 120, 198–203. https://doi.org/10.1016/j.micpath.2018.04.036

340 Mathai, K, Anand, S, Aravind, A, Dinatius, P, Krishnan, AV & Mathai, M. (2017). Antimicrobial Effect of Ginger, Garlic, Honey, and Lemon Extracts on Streptococcus mutans. The Journal of Contemporary Dental Practice, 18(11), 1004–1008. https://doi.org/10.5005/jp-journals-10024-2165

341 de Oliveira, JR, de Jesus, D, Figueira, LW, de Oliveira, FE, Pacheco Soares, C, Camargo, SE, Jorge, AO & de Oliveira, LD. (2017). Biological activities of Rosmarinus officinalis L. (rosemary) extract as analyzed in microorganisms and cells. Experimental Biology and Medicine (Maywood, N.J.), 242(6), 625–634. https://doi.org/10.1177/1535370216688571

342 Młyniec, K, Gaweł, M, Doboszewska, U, Starowicz, G & Nowak, G. (2017). The Role of Elements in Anxiety. Vitamins and Hormones, 103, 295–326. https://doi.org/10.1016/bs.vh.2016.09.002

343 Robinson, DG, Gallego, JA, John, M, Hanna, LA, Zhang, JP, Birnbaum, ML, Greenberg, J, Naraine, M, Peters, BD, McNamara, RK, Malhotra, AK & Szeszko, PR. (2019). A potential role for adjunctive omega-3 polyunsaturated fatty acids for depression and anxiety symptoms in recent onset psychosis: Results from a 16 week randomized placebo-controlled trial for participants concurrently treated with risperidone. Schizophrenia Research, 204, 295–303. https://doi.org/10.1016/j.schres.2018.09.006

344 Zalachoras, I, Hollis, F, Ramos-Fernández, E, Trovo, L, Sonnay, S, Geiser, E, Preitner, N, Steiner, P, Sandi, C & Morató, L. (2020). Therapeutic potential of glutathione-enhancers in stress-related psychopathologies. Neuroscience and Biobehavioral Reviews, 114, 134–155. https://doi.org/10.1016/j.neubiorev.2020.03.015

345 Young, LM, Pipingas, A, White, DJ, Gauci, S & Scholey, A. (2019). A Systematic Review and Meta-Analysis of B Vitamin Supplementation on Depressive Symptoms, Anxiety, and Stress: Effects on Healthy and 'At-Risk' Individuals. Nutrients, 11(9), 2232. https://doi.org/10.3390/nu11092232

346 de Oliveira, IJ, de Souza, VV, Motta, V & Da-Silva, SL. (2015). Effects of Oral Vitamin C Supplementation on Anxiety in Students: A Double-Blind, Randomized, Placebo-Controlled Trial. Pakistan Journal of Biological Sciences PJBS, 18(1), 11–18. https://doi.org/10.3923/pjbs.2015.11.18

347 Eid, A, Khoja, S, AlGhamdi, S, Alsufiani, H, Alzeben, F, Alhejaili, N, Tayeb, HO & Tarazi, FI. (2019). Vitamin D supplementation ameliorates severity of generalized anxiety disorder (GAD). Metabolic Brain Disease, 34(6), 1781–1786. https://doi.org/10.1007/s11011-019-00486-1

348 Roszkowska, A, Pawlicka, M, Mroczek, A, Bałabuszek, K & Nieradko-Iwanicka, B. (2019). Non-Celiac Gluten Sensitivity: A Review. Medicina (Kaunas, Lithuania), 55(6), 222. https://doi.org/10.3390/medicina55060222

349 Sumathi, T, Manivasagam, T & Thenmozhi, AJ. (2020). The Role of Gluten in Autism. Advances in Neurobiology, 24, 469–479. https://doi.org/10.1007/978-3-030-30402-7_14

350 Di Liberto, D, D'Anneo, A, Carlisi, D, Emanuele, S, De Blasio, A, Calvaruso, G, Giuliano, M & Lauricella, M. (2020). Brain Opioid Activity and Oxidative Injury: Different Molecular Scenarios Connecting Celiac Disease and Autistic Spectrum Disorder. Brain Sciences, 10(7), 437. https://doi.org/10.3390/brainsci10070437

351 Trivedi, MS, Shah, JS, Al-Mughairy, S, Hodgson, NW, Simms, B, Trooskens, GA, Van Criekinge, W & Deth, RC. (2014). Food-derived opioid peptides inhibit cysteine uptake with redox and epigenetic consequences. The Journal of Nutritional Biochemistry, 25(10), 1011-1018. https://doi.org/10.1016/j.jnutbio.2014.05.004

352 de Punder, K & Pruimboom, L. (2013). The dietary intake of wheat and other cereal grains and their role in inflammation. Nutrients, 5(3), 771–787. https://doi.org/10.3390/nu5030771

353 Ly, V, Bottelier, M, Hoekstra, PJ, Arias Vasquez, A, Buitelaar, JK & Rommelse, NN. (2017). Elimination diets' efficacy and mechanisms in attention deficit hyperactivity disorder and autism spectrum disorder. European Child & Adolescent Psychiatry, 26(9), 1067–1079. https://doi.org/10.1007/s00787-017-0959-1

354 Hadjivassiliou, M, Aeschlimann, D, Grünewald, RA, Sanders, DS, Sharrack, B & Woodroofe, N. (2011). GAD antibody-associated neurological illness and its relationship to gluten sensitivity. Acta Neurologica Scandinavica, 123(3), 175–180. https://doi.org/10.1111/j.1600-0404.2010.01356.x

355 Thiruvengadam, M, Venkidasamy, B, Thirupathi, P, Chung, IM & Subramanian, U. (2021). β-Casomorphin: A complete health perspective. Food Chemistry, 337, 127765. https://doi.org/10.1016/j.foodchem.2020.127765

356 Garcia-Larsen, V, Ierodiakonou, D, Jarrold, K, Cunha, S, Chivinge, J, Robinson, Z, Geoghegan, N, Ruparelia, A, Devani, P, Trivella, M, Leonardi-Bee, J & Boyle, RJ. (2018). Diet during pregnancy and infancy and risk of allergic or autoimmune disease: A systematic review and meta-analysis. PLoS medicine, 15(2), e1002507. https://doi.org/10.1371/journal.pmed.1002507

357 Lomer, MC. (2015). Review article: the aetiology, diagnosis, mechanisms and clinical evidence for food intolerance. Alimentary Pharmacology & Therapeutics, 41(3), 262–275. https://doi.org/10.1111/apt.13041

358 Jansen, SC, van Dusseldorp, M, Bottema, KC & Dubois, AE. (2003). Intolerance to dietary biogenic amines: a review. Annals of Allergy, Asthma & Immunology: official publication of the American College of Allergy, Asthma, & Immunology, 91(3), 233–296. https://doi.org/10.1016/S1081-1206(10)63523-5

359 Onaolapo, AY & Onaolapo, OJ. (2020). Dietary glutamate and the brain: In the footprints of a Jekyll and Hyde molecule. Neurotoxicology, 80, 93–104. https://doi.org/10.1016/j.neuro.2020.07.001

360 Haroon, E, Miller, AH & Sanacora, G. (2016). Inflammation, glutamate, and glia: A trio of trouble in mood disorders. Neuropsychopharmacology, 42(1), 193-215. https://doi.org/10.1038/npp.2016.199

361 Skypala, IJ, Williams, M, Reeves, L, Meyer, R & Venter, C. (2015). Sensitivity to food additives, vaso-active amines and salicylates: a review of the evidence. Clinical and Translational Allergy, 5, 34. https://doi.org/10.1186/s13601-015-0078-3

362 Huang, Y, Zhang, Y, Chi, Z, Huang, R, Huang, H, Liu, G, Zhang, Y, Yang, H, Lin, J, Yang, T & Cao, S. (2019). The handling of oxalate in the body and the origin of oxalate in calcium oxalate stones. Urologia Internationalis, 104(3-4), 167-176. https://doi.org/10.1159/000504417

363 Lewanika, TR, Reid, SJ, Abratt, VR, Macfarlane, GT & Macfarlane, S. (2007). Lactobacillus gasseri Gasser AM63T degrades oxalate in a multistage continuous culture simulator of the human colonic microbiota. FEMS Microbiology Ecology, 61(1), 110-120. https://doi.org/10.1111/j.1574-6941.2007.00327.x

364 Ferraro PM, Taylor EN, Gambaro G, & Curhan, GC. (2018). Vitamin B6 intake and the risk of incident kidney stones. Urolithiasis. 2018;46(3):265-270. doi:10.1007/s00240-017-0999-5

365 Burgis, JC, Nguyen, K, Park, KT & Cox, K. (2016). Response to strict and liberalized specific carbohydrate diet in pediatric Crohn's disease. World Journal of Gastroenterology, 22(6), 2111–2117. https://doi.org/10.3748/wjg.v22.i6.2111

366 Delaunay-Vagliasindi, S, Seneff, S, Coro, S & Campbell-McBride, N. (2021) GAPS Nutritional Protocol as a treatment for PANDAS: A case study. J Orthomol Med. 36(3)

367 Firth, J, Gangwisch, JE, Borisini, A, Wootton, RE & Mayer, EA. (2020). Food and mood: how do diet and nutrition affect mental wellbeing?. BMJ (Clinical research ed.), 369, m2382. https://doi.org/10.1136/bmj.m2382

368 Calkin, CV & Carandang, CG. (2007). Certain eating disorders may be a neuropsychiatric manifestation of PANDAS: case report. Journal of the Canadian Academy of Child and Adolescent Psychiatry Journal de l'Academie canadienne de psychiatrie de l'enfant et de l'adolescent, 16(3), 132–135.

369 Sigall-Boneh, R, et al. (2017). Research Gaps in Diet and Nutrition in Inflammatory Bowel Disease. A Topical Review by D-ECCO Working Group [Dietitians of ECCO], Journal of Crohn's and Colitis, Volume 11, Issue 12, December 2017, Pages 1407–1419, https://doi.org/10.1093/ecco-jcc/jjx109

370 Toufexis, MD, Hommer, R, Gerardi, DM, et al. (2015). Disordered eating and food restrictions in children with PANDAS/PANS. J Child Adolesc Psychopharmacol. 2015; 25(1): 48-56

Step 3: Symptom-Specific Treatment

Anxiety

371 Amitai, M, Chen, A, Weizman, A & Apter, A. (2015). SSRI-Induced Activation Syndrome in Children and Adolescents—What Is Next? Current Treatment Options in Psychiatry, 2(1), 28-37. doi:10.1007/s40501-015-0034-9

372 Lucchelli, JP & Bertschy, G. (2018). Low-Dose Fluoxetine in Four Children with Autistic Spectrum Disorder Improves Self-Injurious Behavior, ADHD-Like Symptoms, and Irritability. Case Reports in Psychiatry, 2018, 1–4. https://doi.org/10.1155/2018/6278501

373 Cook, EH, Jr, Rowlett, R, Jaselskis, C & Leventhal, BL. (1992). Fluoxetine treatment of children and adults with autistic disorder and mental retardation. Journal of the American Academy of Child and Adolescent Psychiatry, 31(4), 739–745. https://doi.org/10.1097/00004583-199207000-00024

374 Steenen, SA, van Wijk, AJ, van der Heijden, GJ, van Westrhenen, R, de Lange, J & de Jongh, A. (2016). Propranolol for the treatment of anxiety disorders: Systematic review and meta-analysis. Journal of Psychopharmacology (Oxford, England), 30(2), 128–139. https://doi.org/10.1177/0269881115612236

375 Raj, SR, Black, BK, Biaggioni, I, Paranjape, SY, Ramirez, M, Dupont, WD & Robertson, D. (2009). Propranolol decreases tachycardia and improves symptoms in the postural tachycardia syndrome: less is more. Circulation, 120(9), 725–734. https://doi.org/10.1161/CIRCULATIONAHA.108.846501

376 Christiansen, S. (2021, January 27). What Are Adaptogen Herbs? Verywell Health. https://www.verywellhealth.com/what-are-adaptogens-4685073

377 Salve, J, Pate, S, Debnath, K & Langade, D. (2019). Adaptogenic and Anxiolytic Effects of Ashwagandha Root Extract in Healthy Adults: A Double-blind, Randomized, Placebo-controlled Clinical Study. Cureus, 11(12), e6466. https://doi.org/10.7759/cureus.6466

378 Cropley, M, Banks, AP & Boyle, J. (2015). The Effects of Rhodiola rosea L. Extract on Anxiety, Stress, Cognition and Other Mood Symptoms. Phytotherapy research PTR, 29(12), 1934–1939. https://doi.org/10.1002/ptr.5486

379 Ghazizadeh, J, Sadigh-Eteghad, S, Marx, W, Fakhari, A, Hamedeyazdan, S, Torbati, M, Taheri-Tarighi, S, Araj-Khodaei, M, Mirghafourvand, M. (2021). The effects of lemon balm (Melissa officinalis L.) on depression and anxiety in clinical trials: A systematic review and meta-analysis. Phytother Res. 2021 Dec;35(12):6690-6705. doi: 10.1002/ptr.7252.

380 Akhondzadeh, S, Naghavi, HR, Vazirian, M, Shayeganpour, A, Rashidi, H, Khani, M. (2001). Passionflower in the treatment of generalized anxiety: a pilot double-blind randomized controlled trial with oxazepam. J Clin Pharm Ther. 2001 Oct;26(5):363-7. doi: 10.1046/j.1365-2710.2001.00367.x.

381 Jamshidi, N & Cohen, MM. (2017). The Clinical Efficacy and Safety of Tulsi in Humans: A Systematic Review of the Literature. Evidence-based Complementary and Alternative Medicine eCAM, 2017, 9217567. https://doi.org/10.1155/2017/9217567

382 Jin, Z, Kim, S, Cho, S, Kim, IH, Han, D & Jin, YH. (2013). Potentiating effect of glabridin on GABA receptor-mediated responses in dorsal raphe neurons. Planta Medica, 79(15), 1408–1412. https://doi.org/10.1055/s-0033-1350698

383 Lin, B & Li, S. (2011). Cordyceps as an Herbal Drug. In: Benzie IFF, Wachtel-Galor S, editors. Herbal Medicine: Biomolecular and Clinical Aspects. 2nd edition. Boca Raton (FL): CRC Press/Taylor & Francis; 2011. Chapter 5. Available from: www.ncbi.nlm.nih.gov/books/NBK92758/

384 Anderson, S, Panka, J, Rakobitsch, R, Tyre, K & Pulliam, K. (2016). Anxiety and Methylenetetrahydrofolate Reductase Mutation Treated With S-Adenosyl Methionine and Methylated B Vitamins. Integrative Medicine (Encinitas, Calif.), 15(2), 48–52.

385 Rossignol, DA & Frye, RE. (2021). Cerebral Folate Deficiency, Folate Receptor Alpha Autoantibodies and Leucovorin (Folinic Acid) Treatment in Autism Spectrum Disorders: A Systematic Review and Meta-Analysis. Journal of Personalized Medicine, 11(11), 1141. https://doi.org/10.3390/jpm11111141

386 Perli, T, Wronska, AK, Ortiz-Merino, RA, Pronk, JT & Daran, JM. (2020). Vitamin requirements and biosynthesis in Saccharomyces cerevisiae. Yeast (Chichester, England), 37(4), 283–304. https://doi.org/10.1002/yea.3461

387 Mukai, T, Kishi, T, Matsuda, Y & Iwata, N. (2014). A meta-analysis of inositol for depression and anxiety disorders. Human psychopharmacology, 29(1), 55–63. https://doi.org/10.1002/hup.2369

388 Boyle, N, Lawton, C & Dye, L. (2017). The Effects of Magnesium Supplementation on Subjective Anxiety and Stress—A Systematic Review. Nutrients, 9(5), 429. https://doi.org/10.3390/nu9050429

389 Durlach, J, Pagès, N, Bac, P, Bara, M & Guiet-Bara, A. (2004). Magnesium research: from the beginnings to today. Magnesium Research, 17(3), 163–168.

390 Gauthier, I & Nuss, P. (2015). Anxiety disorders and GABA neurotransmission: a disturbance of modulation. Neuropsychiatric Disease and Treatment, 165. https://doi.org/10.2147/ndt.s58841

391 Skelley, JW, Deas, CM, Curren, Z & Ennis, J. (2020). Use of cannabidiol in anxiety and anxiety-related disorders. Journal of the American Pharmacists Association JAPhA, 60(1), 253–261. https://doi.org/10.1016/j.japh.2019.11.008

392 Babaev, O, Piletti Chatain, C & Krueger-Burg, D. (2018). Inhibition in the amygdala anxiety circuitry. Experimental & Molecular Medicine, 50(4), 1–16. https://doi.org/10.1038/s12276-018-0063-8

393 Abdou, AM, Higashiguchi, S, Horie, K, Kim, M, Hatta, H & Yokogoshi, H. (2006). Relaxation and immunity enhancement effects of gamma-aminobutyric acid (GABA) administration in humans. BioFactors (Oxford, England), 26(3), 201–208. https://doi.org/10.1002/biof.5520260305

394 Kim, S, Jo, K, Hong, KB, Han, SH & Suh, HJ. (2019). GABA and l-theanine mixture decreases sleep latency and improves NREM sleep. Pharmaceutical Biology, 57(1), 65–73. https://doi.org/10.1080/13880209.2018.1557698

395 Anderson, E & Shivakumar, G. (2013). Effects of Exercise and Physical Activity on Anxiety. Frontiers in Psychiatry, 4. https://doi.org/10.3389/fpsyt.2013.00027

Tics

396 American Psychiatric Association. (2013). Diagnostic and statistical manual of mental disorders, 5th edition: DSM-5. Washington, DC.

397 Centers for Disease Control and Prevention (CDC). (2009). Prevalence of diagnosed Tourette syndrome in persons aged 6-17 years United States, 2007. MMWR. Morbidity and Mortality Weekly Report, 58(21), 581–585.

398 Xue, W, You, J, Su, Y & Wang, Q. (2019). The Effect of Magnesium Deficiency on Neurological Disorders: A Narrative Review Article. Iranian Journal of Public Health, 48(3), 379–387.

399 Mousain-Bosc, M, Siatka, C & Bali, JP. (2011). Magnesium, hyperactivity and autism in children. In: Vink R, Nechifor M, editors. Magnesium in the Central Nervous System [Internet]. Adelaide (AU): University of Adelaide Press. Available from: https://www.ncbi.nlm.nih.gov/books/NBK507249/

400 Garcia-Lopez, R, Perea-Milla, E, Garcia, CR, Rivas-Ruiz, F, Romero-Gonzalez, J, Moreno, JL, Faus, V, Aguas, G & Diaz, JC. (2009). New therapeutic approach to Tourette Syndrome in children based on a randomized placebo-controlled double-blind phase IV study of the effectiveness and safety of magnesium and vitamin B6. Trials, 10, 16. https://doi.org/10.1186/1745-6215-10-16

401 Koppel, BS. (2015). Cannabis in the Treatment of Dystonia, Dyskinesias, and Tics. Neurotherapeutics: the Journal of the American Society for Experimental NeuroTherapeutics, 12(4), 788–792. https://doi.org/10.1007/s13311-015-0376-4

402 Deepmala, Slattery, J, Kumar, N, Delhey, L, Berk, M, Dean, O, Spielholz, C & Frye, R. (2015). Clinical trials of N-acetylcysteine in psychiatry and neurology: A systematic review. Neuroscience and Biobehavioral Reviews, 55, 294–321. https://doi.org/10.1016/j.neubiorev.2015.04.015

403 Hoffer, ME, Balaban, C, Slade, MD, Tsao, JW & Hoffer, B. (2013). Amelioration of acute sequelae of blast induced mild traumatic brain injury by N-acetyl cysteine: a double-blind, placebo controlled study. PloS one, 8(1), e54163. https://doi.org/10.1371/journal.pone.0054163

404 Draper, A, Stephenson, MC, Jackson, GM, Pépés, S, Morgan, PS, Morris, PG & Jackson, SR. (2014). Increased GABA contributes to enhanced control over motor excitability in Tourette syndrome. Current Biology CB, 24(19), 2343–2347. https://doi.org/10.1016/j.cub.2014.08.038

405 Nathan, PJ, Lu, K, Gray, M & Oliver, C. (2006). The neuropharmacology of L-theanine(N-ethyl-L-glutamine): a possible neuroprotective and cognitive enhancing agent. Journal of Herbal Pharmacotherapy, 6(2), 21–30.

406 Bent, S, Padula, A, Moore, D, Patterson, M & Mehling, W. (2006). Valerian for sleep: a systematic review and meta-analysis. The American Journal of Medicine, 119(12), 1005–1012. https://doi.org/10.1016/j.amjmed.2006.02.026

407 Adib-Hajbaghery, M & Mousavi, SN. (2017). The effects of chamomile extract on sleep quality among elderly people: A clinical trial. Complementary Therapies in Medicine, 35, 109–114. https://doi.org/10.1016/j.ctim.2017.09.010

408 Pringsheim, T, Holler-Managan, Y, Okun, MS, Jankovic, J, Piacentini, J, Cavanna, AE, Martino, D, Müller-Vahl, K, Woods, DW, Robinson, M, Jarvie, E, Roessner, V & Oskoui, M. (2019). Comprehensive systematic review summary: Treatment of tics in people with Tourette syndrome and chronic tic disorders. Neurology, 92(19), 907–915. https://doi.org/10.1212/WNL.0000000000007467

409 Qasaymeh, MM & Mink, JW. (2006). New treatments for tic disorders. Current Treatment Options in Neurology, 8(6), 465–473. https://doi.org/10.1007/s11940-006-0036-4

410 Eddy CM, Rickards HE, Cavanna AE. (2011). Treatment strategies for tics in Tourette syndrome. Ther Adv Neurol Disord. 2011; 4(1): 25-45. doi:10.1177/1756285610390261

411 Read, J & Williams, J. (2019). Positive and Negative Effects of Antipsychotic Medication: An International Online Survey of 832 Recipients. Current Drug Safety, 14(3), 173–181. https://doi.org/10.2174/1574886314666190301152734

412 Martínez-Granero, MA, García-Pérez, A & Montañes, F. Levetiracetam as an alternative therapy for Tourette syndrome. Neuropsychiatr Dis Treat. 2010;6:309-316. Published 2010 Jun 24. doi:10.2147/ndt.s6371

413 Bergeron, R, Ravindran, AV, Chaput, Y, Goldner, E, Swinson, R, Van Ameringen, MA, Austin, C & Hadrava, V. (2002). Sertraline and fluoxetine treatment of obsessive-compulsive disorder: Results of a double-blind, 6-Month treatment study. Journal of Clinical Psychopharmacology, 22(2), 148-154. https://doi.org/10.1097/00004714-200204000-00007

414 Porta, M, Sassi, M, Cavallazzi, M, Fornari, M, Brambilla, A & Servello, D. (2008). Tourette's syndrome and role of tetrabenazine: review and personal experience. Clinical Drug Investigation, 28(7), 443–459. https://doi.org/10.2165/00044011-200828070-00006

415 Pandey, S, Srivanitchapoom, P, Kirubakaran, R & Berman, BD. (2018). Botulinum toxin for motor and phonic tics in Tourette's syndrome. The Cochrane Database of Systematic Reviews, 1(1), CD012285. https://doi.org/10.1002/14651858.CD012285.pub2

416 Sanders, LM & Zeisel, SH. (2007). Choline: Dietary Requirements and Role in Brain Development. Nutrition Today, 42(4), 181–186. https://doi.org/10.1097/01.NT.0000286155.55343.fa

417 Ludlow, AK & Rogers, SL. (2018). Understanding the impact of diet and nutrition on symptoms of Tourette syndrome: A scoping review. Journal of Child Health Care: for Professionals Working with Children in the Hospital and Community, 22(1), 68–83. https://doi.org/10.1177/1367493517748373

418 Jindal, V, Ge, A & Mansky, PJ. (2008). Safety and efficacy of acupuncture in children: a review of the evidence. Journal of Pediatric Hematology/Oncology, 30(6), 431–442. https://doi.org/10.1097/MPH.0b013e318165b2cc

419 Nixon, E, Glazebrook, C, Hollis, C & Jackson, GM. (2014). Reduced Tic Symptomatology in Tourette Syndrome After an Acute Bout of Exercise: An Observational Study. Behavior Modification, 38(2), 235–263. https://doi.org/10.1177/0145445514532127

420 Nosratmirshekarlou, E, Shafiq, S, Goodarzi, ZS, Martino, D & Pringsheim, T. (2019). Effect of diet, exercise and sleep on tic severity: a scoping review protocol. BMJ Open, 9(7), e024653. https://doi.org/10.1136/bmjopen-2018-024653

Obsessive-Compulsive Disorder (OCD)

421 American Psychiatric Association. Diagnostic and statistical manual of mental disorders, 5th edition: DSM-5. Washington, DC; 2013.

422 Gerentes, M, Pelissolo, A, Rajagopal, K, Tamouza, R & Hamdani, N. (2019). Obsessive-Compulsive Disorder: Autoimmunity and Neuroinflammation. Current Psychiatry Reports, 21(8), 78. https://doi.org/10.1007/s11920-019-1062-8

423 Chang, K, Frankovich, J, Cooperstock, M, et al. (2015). Clinical evaluation of youth with pediatric acute-onset neuropsychiatric syndrome (PANS): recommendations from the 2013 PANS Consensus Conference. J. Child Adolesc. Psychopharmacol 25(1), 3-13.

424 Pittenger, C & Bloch, MH. (2014). Pharmacological treatment of obsessive-compulsive disorder. Psychiatr Clin North Am. 2014; 37(3): 375-391. doi:10.1016/j.psc.2014.05.006

425 Kaurav, BP, Wanjari, MM, Chandekar, A, Chauhan, NS & Upmanyu, N. (2012). Influence of Withania somnifera on obsessive compulsive disorder in mice. Asian Pacific Journal of Tropical Medicine, 5(5), 380–384. https://doi.org/10.1016/S1995-7645(12)60063-7

426 Javadian, F, Sepehri, Z, Saeidi, S & Hassanshahian, M. (2017). Antifungal effects of the extract of the Withania somnifera on Candida albicans. Advanced Herbal Medicine, 3(1), 31-37.

427 Salve, J, Pate, S, Debnath, K & Langade, D. (2019). Adaptogenic and Anxiolytic Effects of Ashwagandha Root Extract in Healthy Adults: A Double-blind, Randomized, Placebo-controlled Clinical Study. Cureus, 11(12), e6466. https://doi.org/10.7759/cureus.6466

428 Janda, K, Wojtkowska, K, Jakubczyk, K, Antoniewicz, J & Skonieczna-Żydecka, K. (2020). Passiflora incarnata in Neuropsychiatric Disorders-A Systematic Review. Nutrients, 12(12), 3894. https://doi.org/10.3390/nu12123894

429 Akhondzadeh, S, Naghavi, HR, Vazirian, M, Shayeganpour, A, Rashidi, H & Khani, M. (2001). Passionflower in the treatment of generalized anxiety: a pilot double-blind randomized controlled trial with oxazepam. Journal of Clinical Pharmacy and Therapeutics, 26(5), 363–367. https://doi.org/10.1046/j.1365-2710.2001.00367.x

430 Mauzay, D, LaFrance, EM & Cuttler, C. (2021). Acute Effects of Cannabis on Symptoms of Obsessive-Compulsive Disorder. Journal of Affective Disorders, 279, 158–163. https://doi.org/10.1016/j.jad.2020.09.124

431 Nardo, M, Casarotto, PC, Gomes, FV & Guimarães, FS. (2014). Cannabidiol reverses the mCPP-induced increase in marble-burying behavior. Fundamental & Clinical Pharmacology, 28(5), 544–550. https://doi.org/10.1111/fcp.12051

432 di Michele, F, Siracusano, A, Talamo, A & Niolu, C. (2018). N-Acetyl Cysteine and Vitamin D Supplementation in Treatment Resistant Obsessive-compulsive Disorder Patients: A General Review. Current Pharmaceutical Design, 24(17), 1832–1838. https://doi.org/10.2174/1381612824666180417124919

433 Rodrigues-Barata, AR, Tosti, A, Rodríguez-Pichardo, A & Camacho-Martínez, F. (2012). N-acetylcysteine in the Treatment of Trichotillomania. International Journal of Trichology, 4(3), 176–178. https://doi.org/10.4103/0974-7753.100090

434 Grant, JE, Kim, SW & Odlaug, BL. (2007). N-acetyl cysteine, a glutamate-modulating agent, in the treatment of pathological gambling: a pilot study. Biological Psychiatry, 62(6), 652–657. https://doi.org/10.1016/j.biopsych.2006.11.021

435 Berk, M, Jeavons, S, Dean, OM, Dodd, S, Moss, K, Gama, CS & Malhi, GS. (2009). Nail-biting stuff? The effect of N-acetyl cysteine on nail-biting. CNS Spectrums, 14(7), 357–360. https://doi.org/10.1017/s1092852900023002

436 Grant, JE, Chamberlain, SR, Redden, SA, Leppink, EW, Odlaug, BL & Kim, SW. (2016). N-Acetylcysteine in the Treatment of Excoriation Disorder: A Randomized Clinical Trial. JAMA Psychiatry, 73(5), 490–496. https://doi.org/10.1001/jamapsychiatry.2016.0060

437 Fux, M, Levine, J, Aviv, A & Belmaker, RH. (1996). Inositol treatment of obsessive-compulsive disorder. The American Journal of Psychiatry, 153(9), 1219–1221. https://doi.org/10.1176/ajp.153.9.1219

438 Maffei, ME. (2020). 5-Hydroxytryptophan (5-HTP): Natural Occurrence, Analysis, Biosynthesis, Biotechnology, Physiology and Toxicology. International Journal of Molecular Sciences, 22(1), 181. https://doi.org/10.3390/ijms22010181

439 Greenblatt, JM. (2016). Nutritional Lithium: A Cinderella Story: The Untold Tale of a Mineral That Transforms Lives and Heals the Brain..

440 Dwivedi, T & Zhang, H. (2014). Lithium-induced neuroprotection is associated with epigenetic modification of specific BDNF gene promoter and altered apoptotic-regulatory proteins. Front Neurosci 8:1-8.

441 Russo, AJ & Pietsch, SC. (2013). Decreased Hepatocyte Growth Factor (HGF) and Gamma Aminobutyric Acid (GABA) in Individuals with Obsessive-Compulsive Disorder (OCD). Biomarker Insights, 8, 107–114. https://doi.org/10.4137/BMI.S11931

442 Botturi, A, Ciappolino, V, Delvecchio, G, Boscutti, A, Viscardi, B & Brambilla, P. (2020). The Role and the Effect of Magnesium in Mental Disorders: A Systematic Review. Nutrients, 12(6), 1661. https://doi.org/10.3390/nu12061661

443 Sayyah, M, Olapour, A, Saeedabad, YS, Yazdan Parast, R & Malayeri, A. (2012). Evaluation of oral zinc sulfate effect on obsessive-compulsive disorder: a randomized placebo-controlled clinical trial. Nutrition (Burbank, Los Angeles County, Calif.), 28(9), 892–895. https://doi.org/10.1016/j.nut.2011.11.027

444 Masand, PS, Keuthen, NJ, Gupta, S, Virk, S, Yu-Siao, B & Kaplan, D. (2006). Prevalence of irritable bowel syndrome in obsessive-compulsive disorder. CNS Spectrums, 11(1), 21–25. https://doi.org/10.1017/s1092852900024123

445 Lakhan, SE & Vieira, KF. (2008). Nutritional therapies for mental disorders. Nutrition Journal, 7, 2. https://doi.org/10.1186/1475-2891-7-2

Brain Fog

446 Murphy, TK, Patel, PD, McGuire, JF, Kennel, A, Mutch, PJ, Parker-Athill, EC, Hanks, CE, Lewin, AB, Storch, EA, Toufexis, MD, Dadlani, GH & Rodriguez, CA. (2015). "Characterization of the pediatric acute-onset neuropsychiatric syndrome phenotype." J Child Adolesc Psychopharmacol. 2015 Feb; 25(1): 14-25. doi: 10.1089/cap.2014.0062. Epub 2014 Oct 14.

447 Toufexis, MD, Hommer, R, Gerardi, DM, Grant, P, Rothschild, L, D'Souza, P, Williams, K, Leckman, J, Swedo, SE & Murphy, TK. (2015). Disordered eating and food restrictions in children with PANDAS/PANS. Journal of Child and Adolescent Psychopharmacology, 25(1), 48–56. https://doi.org/10.1089/cap.2014.0063

448 Swanson, CJ, Perry, KW, Koch-Krueger, S, Katner, J, Svensson, KA & Bymaster, FP. (2006). Effect of the attention deficit/hyperactivity disorder drug atomoxetine on extracellular concentrations of norepinephrine and dopamine in several brain regions of the rat. Neuropharmacology, 50(6), 755–760. https://doi.org/10.1016/j.neuropharm.2005.11.022

449 Strawn, JR, Compton, SN, Robertson, B, Albano, AM, Hamdani, M & Rynn, MA. (2017). Extended Release Guanfacine in Pediatric Anxiety Disorders: A Pilot, Randomized, Placebo-Controlled Trial. Journal of Child and Adolescent Psychopharmacology, 27(1), 29–37. https://doi.org/10.1089/cap.2016.0132

450 Russo, A & Borrelli, F. (2005). Bacopa monniera, a reputed nootropic plant: an overview. Phytomedicine, 12(4), 305–317. https://doi.org/10.1016/j.phymed.2003.12.008

Sleep

451 Gaughan, T, Buckley, A, Hommer, R, Grant, P, Williams, K, Leckman, JF & Swedo, SE. (2016). Rapid Eye Movement Sleep Abnormalities in Children with Pediatric Acute-Onset Neuropsychiatric Syndrome (PANS). Journal of Clinical Sleep Medicine JCSM official publication of the American Academy of Sleep Medicine, 12(7), 1027–1032. https://doi.org/10.5664/jcsm.5942

452 Goldstein, AN, Greer, SM, Saletin, JM, Harvey, AG, Nitschke, JB & Walker, MP. (2013). Tired and apprehensive: anxiety amplifies the impact of sleep loss on aversive brain anticipation. The Journal of Neuroscience: the Official Journal of the Society for Neuroscience, 33(26), 10607–10615. https://doi.org/10.1523/JNEUROSCI.5578-12.2013

453 Eugene, AR & Masiak, J. (2015). The Neuroprotective Aspects of Sleep. MEDtube Science, 3(1), 35–40.

454 Savarese, M, Carnicelli, M, Cardinali, V, Mogavero, MP & Federico, F. (2015). Subjective hypnotic efficacy of Trazodone and Mirtazapine in patients with chronic insomnia: a retrospective, comparative study. Archives Italiennes de Biologie, 153(2-3), 231–238. https://doi.org/10.12871/0003982920152348

455 Aulinas, A. (2019). Physiology of the Pineal Gland and Melatonin. In K. R. Feingold (Eds.) et. al., Endotext. MDText.com, Inc.

456 Ferracioli-Oda, E, Qawasmi, A & Bloch, MH. (2013). Meta-analysis: melatonin for the treatment of primary sleep disorders. PloS one, 8(5), e63773. https://doi.org/10.1371/journal.pone.0063773

457 Rios, P, Cardoso, R, Morra, D, et al. (2019). Comparative effectiveness and safety of pharmacological and non-pharmacological interventions for insomnia: an overview of reviews. Syst Rev 8, 281. https://doi.org/10.1186/s13643-019-1163-9

458 Pugle, M. (2021, March 18). GABA: What It Is, Functions, and Disorders. Verywell Health. www.verywellhealth.com/gaba-5095143

459 Juneja, L, Chu, D, Ōkubo, T, Nagato, Y & Yokogoshi, H. (1999). L-theanine—a unique amino acid of green tea and its relaxation effect in humans. Trends in Food Science and Technology, 10, 199-204.

460 Hong, KB, Park, Y & Suh, HJ. (2018). Two combined amino acids promote sleep activity in caffeine-induced sleepless model systems. Nutrition Research and Practice, 12(3), 208–214. https://doi.org/10.4162/nrp.2018.12.3.208

461 Breus, M. (2018, May 14). What You Need to Know About Magnesium and Your Sleep. Psychology Today. www.psychologytoday.com/us/blog/sleep-newzzz/201805/what-you-need-know-about-magnesium-and-your-sleep

462 Gagliano, A, Puligheddu, M, Ronzano, N, Congiu, P, Tanca, MG, Cursio, I, Carucci, S, Sotgiu, S, Grossi, E & Zuddas, A. (2021). Artificial Neural Networks Analysis of polysomnographic and clinical features in Pediatric Acute-Onset Neuropsychiatric Syndrome (PANS): from sleep alteration to "Brain Fog". Nature and Science of Sleep, 13, 1209–1224. https://doi.org/10.2147/NSS.S300818

Constipation

463 Tabbers, MM, DiLorenzo, C, Berger, MY, Faure, C, Langendam, MW, Nurko, S, Staiano, A, Vandenplas, Y & Benninga, MA European Society for Pediatric Gastroenterology, Hepatology, and Nutrition; North American Society for Pediatric Gastroenterology. (2014). Evaluation and treatment of functional constipation in infants and children: evidence-based recommendations from ESPGHAN and NASPGHAN. J Pediatr Gastroenterol Nutr. 2014 Feb; 58(2): 258-74. doi: 10.1097/MPG.0000000000000266.

464 Ferguson, BJ, Marler, S, Altstein, LL, Lee, EB, Akers, J, Sohl, K, McLaughlin, A, Hartnett, K, Kille, B, Mazurek, M, Macklin, EA, McDonnell, E, Barstow, M, Bauman, ML, Margolis, KG, Veenstra-VanderWeele, J & Beversdorf, DQ. (2017). Psychophysiological Associations with Gastrointestinal Symptomatology in Autism Spectrum Disorder. Autism Research: Official Journal of the International Society for Autism Research, 10(2), 276–288. https://doi.org/10.1002/aur.1646

465 Peters, B, Williams, KC, Gorrindo, P, et al. (2014). Rigid-compulsive behaviors are associated with mixed bowel symptoms in autism spectrum disorder. J Autism Dev Disord. 2014; 44(6): 1425-1432.

466 Paré, P, Bridges, R, Champion, MC, Ganguli, SC, Gray, JR, Irvine, EJ, Plourde, V, Poitras, P, Turnbull, GK, Moayyedi, P, Flook, N & Collins, SM. (2007). Recommendations on chronic constipation (including constipation associated with irritable bowel syndrome) treatment. Canadian Journal of Gastroenterology = Journal Canadien de Gastroenterologie, 21 Suppl B(Suppl B), 3B–22B.

467 Ellis, E. (2020, November 3). Fiber. Eat Right. www.eatright.org

468 Tresca, A. (2021, September 24). Discover the Benefits, Side Effects, and Dosage of Magnesium Citrate. Verywell Health. www.verywellhealth.com/magnesium-citrate-benefits-side-effects-dosage-and-interactions-4177658

469 el Baza, F, AlShahawi, HA, Zahra, S & AbdelHakim, RA. (2016). Magnesium supplementation in children with attention deficit hyperactivity disorder. Egyptian Journal of Medical Human Genetics, 17(1), 63–70. https://doi.org/10.1016/j.ejmhg.2015.05.008

470 Garcia-Lopez, R, Perea-Milla, E, Garcia, CR, Rivas-Ruiz, F, Romero-Gonzalez, J, Moreno, JL, Faus, V, Aguas, GDC & Diaz, JCR. (2009). New therapeutic approach to Tourette Syndrome in children based on a randomized placebo-controlled double-blind phase IV study of the effectiveness and safety of magnesium and vitamin B6. Trials, 10(1). https://doi.org/10.1186/1745-6215-10-16

471 Hong, SW, Chun, J, Park, S, Lee, HJ, Im, JP & Kim, JS. (2018). Aloe vera Is Effective and Safe in Short-term Treatment of Irritable Bowel Syndrome: A Systematic Review and Meta-analysis. Journal of Neurogastroenterology and Motility, 24(4), 528–535. https://doi.org/10.5056/jnm18077

472 Langmead, L, Makins, RJ & Rampton, DS. (2004). Anti-inflammatory effects of aloe vera gel in human colorectal mucosa in vitro. Alimentary Pharmacology & Therapeutics, 19(5), 521–527. https://doi.org/10.1111/j.1365-2036.2004.01874.x

473 NHS website. (2021, October 6). Senna. Nhs.Uk. https://www.nhs.uk/medicines/senna/

474 Murata, S, Inoue, K, Aomatsu, T, Yoden, A & Tamai, H. (2017). Supplementation with carnitine reduces the severity of constipation: a retrospective study of patients with severe motor and intellectual disabilities. Journal of Clinical Biochemistry and Nutrition, 60(2), 121–124. https://doi.org/10.3164/jcbn.16-52

475 Forootan, M, Bagheri, N & Darvishi, M. (2018). Chronic constipation: A review of literature. Medicine, 97(20), e10631. https://doi.org/10.1097/MD.0000000000010631

Neurotherapy

476 Ozza, A. (2017). Cognitive behavioral therapy and acceptance and commitment therapy as augmentation treatment for paediatric autoimmune neuropsychiatric disorders associated with Streptococcal infections (PANDAS): A case report. European Psychiatry, 41(S1), s781-s782. https://doi.org/10.1016/j.eurpsy.2017.01.1488

477 Hofmann, SG, Asnaani, A, Vonk, IJ, Sawyer, AT & Fang A. (2012) The efficacy of cognitive behavioral therapy: A review of meta-analyses. Cognit Ther Res. 2012; 36(5): 427-440. doi:10.1007/s10608-012-9476-1

478 Artiran, M. (2019). A cross-cultural redefinition of rational emotive and cognitive behavior therapy: From the West to the Middle East. New York, NY: Routledge.

479 Piacentini, J, Wu, M, Rozenman, M, Bennett, S, McGuire, J, Nadeau, J, Lewin, A, Sookman, D, Lindsey Bergman, R, Storch, EA & Peris, T. (2021). Knowledge and competency standards for specialized cognitive behavior therapy for pediatric obsessive-compulsive disorder. Psychiatry Research, 299, 113854. https://doi.org/10.1016/j.psychres.2021.113854

480 Nadeau, JM, et al. (2015). "A pilot trial of cognitive-behavioral therapy augmentation of antibiotic treatment in youth with pediatric acute-onset neuropsychiatric syndrome-related obsessive-compulsive disorder." Journal of child and adolescent psychopharmacology vol. 25, 4: 337-43. doi:10.1089/cap.2014.0149

481 Arnold, LE, Lofthouse, N, Hersch, S, Pan, X, Hurt, E, Bates, B, Kassouf, K, Moone, S & Grantier, C. (2012). EEG Neurofeedback for ADHD. Journal of Attention Disorders, 17(5), 410-419. https://doi.org/10.1177/1087054712446173

482 Wang, B, et al. (2021). EEG-Based Closed-Loop Neurofeedback for Attention Monitoring and Training in Young Adults. Journal of Healthcare Engineering, vol. 2021, Article ID 5535810, 13 pages, 2021. https://doi.org/10.1155/2021/5535810

483 Sürmeli, T & Ertem, A. (2011). Obsessive compulsive disorder and the efficacy of qeeg-guided Neurofeedback treatment: A case series. Clinical EEG and Neuroscience, 42(3), 195-201. https://doi.org/10.1177/155005941104200310

484 Lofthouse, N, Arnold, LE, Hersch, S, Hurt, E & DeBeus, R. (2011). A review of Neurofeedback treatment for pediatric ADHD. Journal of Attention Disorders, 16(5), 351-372. https://doi.org/10.1177/1087054711427530

485 Keng, SL, Smoski, MJ & Robins, CJ. (2011). Effects of mindfulness on psychological health: a review of empirical studies. Clinical Psychology Review, 31(6), 1041–1056. https://doi.org/10.1016/j.cpr.2011.04.006

486 Behan, C. (2020). The benefits of meditation and mindfulness practices during times of crisis such as COVID-19. Irish Journal of Psychological Medicine, 37(4), 256–258. https://doi.org/10.1017/ipm.2020.38

487 Sharma, A, Madaan, V & Petty, FD. (2006). Exercise for mental health. Primary Care Companion to the Journal of Clinical Psychiatry, 8(2), 106. https://doi.org/10.4088/pcc.v08n0208a

488 Smits, JA, Tart, CD, Rosenfield, D & Zvolensky, MJ. (2011). The interplay between physical activity and anxiety sensitivity in fearful responding to carbon dioxide challenge. Psychosomatic Medicine, 73(6), 498–503. https://doi.org/10.1097/PSY.0b013e3182223b28

Case Studies

PANDAS and Mold: Hannah

489 Hope, J. (2013). A review of the mechanism of injury and treatment approaches for illness resulting from exposure to water-damaged buildings, mold, and mycotoxins. The Scientific World Journal, 2013, 767482. https://doi.org/10.1155/2013/767482

OCD/POTS: Kristen

490 Stewart, JM, Boris, JR, Chelimsky, G, Fischer, PR, Fortunato, JE, Grubb, BP, Heyer, GL, Jarjour, IT, Medow, MS, Numan, MT, Pianosi, PT, Singer, W, Tarbell, S, Chelimsky, TC & Pediatric Writing Group of the American Autonomic Society. (2018). Pediatric Disorders of Orthostatic Intolerance. Pediatrics, 141(1), e20171673. https://doi.org/10.1542/peds.2017-1673

491 Xu, WR, Jin, HF & Du, JB. (2016). Pathogenesis and Individualized Treatment for Postural Tachycardia Syndrome in Children. Chinese Medical Journal, 129(18), 2241–2245. https://doi.org/10.4103/0366-6999.189915

492 Pektas, A, Koken, R & Koca, HB. (2018). Serum vitamin B-12 in children presenting with vasovagal syncope. Asia Pacific Journal of Clinical Nutrition, 27(1), 176–181. https://doi.org/10.6133/apjcn.022017.17

Tics and Antioxidants: Caleb

493 Kang, SG, Lee, HJ, Choi, JE, An, H, Rhee, M & Kim, L. (2009). Association study between glutathione S-transferase GST-M1, GST-T1, and GST-P1 polymorphisms and tardive dyskinesia. Human Psychopharmacology, 24(1), 55–60. https://doi.org/10.1002/hup.988

494 Wang, HL, Zhang, J, Li, YP, Dong, L & Chen, YZ. (2021). Potential use of glutathione as a treatment for Parkinson's disease. Experimental and Therapeutic Medicine, 21(2), 125. https://doi.org/10.3892/etm.2020.9557

PANS and COVID: Layla

495 Keller, E, Brandi, G, Winklhofer, S, Imbach, LL, Kirschenbaum, D, Frontzek, K, Steiger, P, Dietler, S, Haeberlin, M, Willms, J, Porta, F, Waeckerlin, A, Huber, M, Abela, IA, Lutterotti, A, Stippich, C, Globas, C, Varga, Z & Jelcic, I. (2020). Large and Small Cerebral Vessel Involvement in Severe COVID-19: Detailed Clinical Workup of a Case Series. Stroke, 51(12), 3719–3722. https://doi.org/10.1161/STROKEAHA.120.031224

496 Rahimi, K. (2020). Guillain-Barre syndrome during COVID-19 pandemic: an overview of the reports. Neurological Sciences: Official Journal of the Italian Neurological Society and of the Italian Society of Clinical Neurophysiology, 41(11), 3149–3156. https://doi.org/10.1007/s10072-020-04693-y

497 Pavone, P, Ceccarelli, M, Marino, S, Caruso, D, Falsaperla, R, Berretta, M, Rullo, EV & Nunnari, G. (2021). SARS-CoV-2 related paediatric acute-onset neuropsychiatric syndrome. The Lancet. Child & Adolescent Health, 5(6), e19–e21. https://doi.org/10.1016/S2352-4642(21)00135-8

498 Merad, M, Subramanian, A & Wang, TT. (2021). An aberrant inflammatory response in severe COVID-19. Cell Host & Microbe, 29(7), 1043–1047. https://doi.org/10.1016/j.chom.2021.06.018

Made in United States
North Haven, CT
15 September 2023

41599461R00204